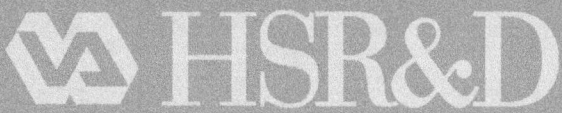

I0470876

Brief Psychotherapy for Depression in Primary Care: A Systematic Review of the Evidence

January 2011

Prepared for:

Department of Veterans Affairs
Veterans Health Administration
Health Services Research & Development Service
Washington, DC 20420

Prepared by:

Evidence-based Synthesis Program (ESP) Center
Durham VA Medical Center
Durham, NC
John W. Williams Jr., MD, MHSc, Director

Investigators:

Principal Investigator:
Jason A. Nieuwsma, PhD

Co-Investigators:
Ranak B. Trivedi, PhD
Jennifer McDuffie, PhD
Ian Kronish, MD
Dinesh Benjamin, MD
John W. Williams Jr., MD, MHSc

Medical Editor:
Liz Wing, MA

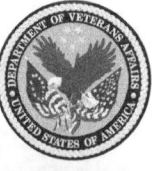

To Contents

PREFACE

Health Services Research & Development Service's (HSR&D's) Evidence-based Synthesis Program (ESP) was established to provide timely and accurate syntheses of targeted healthcare topics of particular importance to Veterans Affairs (VA) managers and policymakers, as they work to improve the health and healthcare of Veterans. The ESP disseminates these reports throughout the VA.

HSR&D provides funding for four ESP Centers and each Center has an active VA affiliation. The ESP Centers generate evidence syntheses on important clinical practice topics, and these reports help:

- develop clinical policies informed by evidence,
- guide the implementation of effective services to improve patient outcomes and to support VA clinical practice guidelines and performance measures, and
- set the direction for future research to address gaps in clinical knowledge.

In 2009, an ESP Coordinating Center was created to expand the capacity of HSR&D Central Office and the four ESP sites by developing and maintaining program processes. In addition, the Center established a Steering Committee comprised of HSR&D field-based investigators, VA Patient Care Services, Office of Quality and Performance, and Veterans Integrated Service Networks (VISN) Clinical Management Officers. The Steering Committee provides program oversight, guides strategic planning, coordinates dissemination activities, and develops collaborations with VA leadership to identify new ESP topics of importance to Veterans and the VA healthcare system.

Comments on this evidence report are welcome and can be sent to Nicole Floyd, ESP Coordinating Center Program Manager, at nicole.floyd@va.gov.

Recommended citation: Nieuwsma JA, Trivedi RB, McDuffie J, Kronish I, Benjamin D, Williams JW Jr. Brief Psychotherapy for Depression in Primary Care: A Systematic Review of the Evidence. VA-ESP Project #09-010; 2011

TABLE OF CONTENTS

FIGURES

TABLES

EXECUTIVE SUMMARY

BACKGROUND

The individual and societal burden of depressive disorders is widely acknowledged, but treating these disorders remains challenging. Clinical guidelines recommend that both pharmacotherapy and psychotherapy should be considered as first-line treatments. Yet, because primary care settings are often the frontline of treatment, pharmacological treatments take precedence. In part, this may be due to the perception that psychotherapy is lengthy and time intensive, with guidelines recommending 12 to 20 1-hour sessions for most evidence-based psychotherapies. However, recent evidence seems to suggest that psychotherapies that are briefer in both duration and intensity may be efficacious in acute-phase treatment. If true, these briefer psychotherapies may be more easily integrated in primary care settings. Thus, we conducted a systematic review of the peer-reviewed literature to answer the following key questions:

Key Question 1: For primary care patients with depressive disorders, are brief, evidence-based psychotherapies with durations of up to eight sessions more efficacious than control for depressive symptoms (i.e., on self-report and/or clinician-administered measures) and quality of life (i.e., functional status and/or health-related quality of life)?

Key Question 2: For primary care patients with depressive disorders treated with a brief, evidence-based psychotherapy, is there evidence that treatment effect may vary by the number of sessions delivered?

Key Question 3: For psychotherapies demonstrating clinically significant treatment effects, what are the characteristics of treatment providers (i.e., type of provider and training), and what are the modalities of therapy (i.e., individual/group, face-to-face/teletherapy/Internet-based)?

Key Question 4: How commonly reported are the key clinical outcomes of quality of life, social functioning, occupational status, patient satisfaction, and adverse treatment effects in randomized trials of psychotherapy?

This review was commissioned by the Department of Veterans Affairs' Evidence-based Synthesis Program. The topic was selected after a formal topic nomination and prioritization process that included representatives from the Office of Mental Health Services, Health Services Research and Development, the Mental Health QUERI, and the Office of Mental Health and Primary Care Integration.

METHODS

We utilized a combined approach, identifying and evaluating existing systematic reviews and supplementing these reviews by searching for and evaluating original research not included in these reviews. First, we searched for relevant, good-quality, English-language systematic reviews in MEDLINE® (via PubMed®), Embase®, and PsycINFO® from database inception through May 2010. Two good-quality systematic reviews were identified and evaluated for this report. Second, we used a well-documented Internet-accessible database of psychotherapy trials (www.psychotherapyrcts.org/index.php?id=3) that was current through January 2010. We used this database of 243 trials as a data source for original research, searching for studies coded as including adults with a mood disorder who received face-to-face psychotherapy at a dose of eight or fewer therapy sessions. Finally, we searched for English-language publications in MEDLINE (via PubMed), PsycINFO, and Embase, from January 2009 (one year prior to the search date of the online database) through August 1, 2010. We supplemented electronic searching by examining the bibliographies of included studies and review articles.

Primary research articles were included if they were RCTs and included adults with major depressive disorder (MDD), dysthymic disorder, or subthreshold (minor) depressive disorder in acute-phase treatment. Relevant psychotherapy modalities included cognitive behavioral therapy (CBT) (including cognitive therapy and behavior therapy), interpersonal therapy (IPT), problem-solving therapy (PST), mindfulness-based cognitive therapy (MBCT), cognitive behavioral analysis system of psychotherapy (CBASP), dialectical behavioral therapy (DBT), functional analytic psychotherapy (FAP), acceptance and commitment therapy (ACT), or short-term psychodynamic therapy with eight or fewer planned sessions. Eligible comparators of active treatment included waitlist control, attention control, usual care, or antidepressant medication if the intervention included a combination of psychotherapy and an antidepressant medication. Patients had to be recruited from outpatient general medical or mental health clinics located in North America, Western Europe, New Zealand, or Australia for the greatest generalizability to the Veteran population. Finally, RCTs were required to measure depressive symptoms using a validated instrument reported at 6 weeks or more after randomization.

Quality of the systematic reviews was rated using 12 design-and-reporting characteristics and summarized as "good," "fair," or "poor." Quality and risk of bias of the RCTs were rated good, fair, or poor using the Agency for Healthcare Research and Quality (AHRQ) criteria. Data were synthesized both in narrative form and via updated meta-analysis where it appeared that the primary literature was sufficient to facilitate an updated effect size. All results are reported such that a negative effect size indicates greater reduction in depressive symptoms for the intervention compared to the control condition. We graded the strength of evidence for each key question using principles from the Grades of Recommendation, Assessment, Development, and Evaluation (GRADE) Working Group. This approach assesses the strength of evidence for each critical outcome by considering risk of bias, consistency, directness, precision, and publication bias. Other domains relevant to observational designs were not pertinent to our review. After considering each domain, a summary rating of "high," "moderate," "low," or "insufficient" strength of evidence was assigned.

RESULTS

Using the combined literature search, 560 potential systematic reviews were identified. From these, two eligible reviews were retained. The first review completed a good-quality meta-analysis of 15 studies that examined psychotherapeutic interventions for depression in primary care. The second review completed a good-quality meta-analysis and meta-regression of 34 studies examining the effectiveness of brief psychological therapies in primary care for anxiety disorders, depressive disorders, and mixed anxiety and depression.

Our search of the primary literature yielded 243 references from the Internet-accessible database of psychotherapy trials and 516 citations from the search of PubMed, PsycINFO, and Embase. After excluding ineligible articles, our search identified eight unique trials from the two included systematic reviews and seven unique trials from our primary literature search. The brief therapies evaluated were PST (eight studies), CBT (six studies), and MBCT (one study). Interventions were monitored for treatment fidelity in nine studies. Study participants were predominantly middle-aged, female, and Caucasian.

Key Question 1: For primary care patients with depressive disorders, are brief, evidence-based psychotherapies with durations of up to eight sessions more efficacious than control for depressive symptoms (i.e., on self-report and/or clinician-administered measures) and quality of life (i.e., functional status and/or health-related quality of life)?

The systematic reviews found that, compared to control, brief psychotherapies had a small but statistically significant benefit, with effect size estimates ranging from -0.33 to -0.25. Only CBT and PST were evaluated as brief therapies. Findings from the systematic reviews were consistent with the meta-analysis that we conducted on six trials of CBT, which showed that six to eight CBT sessions were more efficacious than control (ES -0.42, 95% CI -074 to -0.10), but results were statistically heterogeneous (I^2 = 56%). A sensitivity analysis excluding a poor-quality study and one with a waitlist control showed homogeneous but smaller treatment effects (ES -0.24, 95% CI -0.42 to -0.06, I^2 = 0%). Health-related quality of life (HRQOL) was reported too infrequently to synthesize quantitatively.

Key Question 2: For primary care patients with depressive disorders treated with a brief, evidence-based psychotherapy, is there evidence that treatment effect may vary by the number of sessions delivered?

One of the systematic reviews completed a meta-analysis showing no statistically significant difference in efficacy between psychotherapies of more than six sessions (ES -0.36, 95% CI -0.54 to -0.17) compared to those of six or fewer sessions (ES -0.25, 95% CI -0.48 to -0.02). Because confidence intervals overlapped and comparisons were indirect, there remains the possibility that a true difference in efficacy between brief and standard-duration psychotherapies (i.e., 12 to 20 sessions) could exist and that it could be clinically meaningful. Current evidence is inadequate to answer this question.

Key Question 3: For psychotherapies demonstrating clinically significant treatment effects, what are the characteristics of treatment providers (i.e., type of provider and training), and what are the modalities of therapy (i.e., individual/group, face-to-face/teletherapy/Internet-based)?

Treatment providers and modalities varied across studies. Providers included clinical psychologists, social workers, nurses, general practitioners, and graduate students trained specifically to deliver the treatment as prescribed in the study protocol. Length of treatment varied from 3.5 hours of PST (delivered across six sessions) to 18 hours of MBCT (delivered across eight sessions). Finally, treatments were delivered primarily in individual, face-to-face sessions; however, two studies relied on group therapy, and one trial relied on telephone-based psychotherapy.

Key Question 4: How commonly reported are the key clinical outcomes of quality of life, social functioning, occupational status, patient satisfaction, and adverse treatment effects in randomized trials of psychotherapy?

Of the 15 RCTs evaluating brief psychotherapies, 5 reported HRQOL, 5 reported social functioning, 0 reported occupational status, 2 reported patient satisfaction with treatment, and 1 reported adverse treatment effects. The most commonly used measure of quality of life for studies that examined this clinical outcome was the SF-36. The one study that reported adverse treatment effects examined the side effects of taking psychotropic medication in tandem with psychotherapy.

FUTURE RESEARCH RECOMMENDATIONS

Several questions may be answered by future studies. First, brief psychotherapies (i.e., $\leq$ 8 sessions) compared to standard-duration psychotherapies (i.e., 12 to 20 sessions) did not significantly differ in their effect sizes, but these comparisons were based on relatively few studies and indirect comparisons, and thus direct comparisons in RCTs would be needed to answer this question definitively. Second, our review found that brief psychotherapies have been provided by an array of trained health care professionals, including non–mental health professionals. Because descriptions of training were incomplete, the degree of training necessary to replicate findings from these studies is uncertain. Third, we discovered that effects on occupational status, patient satisfaction with treatment, and adverse treatment effects were seldom reported; HRQOL and social functioning were more commonly reported but still only considered in less than half the trials examined in this review. Therefore, future research should aim to include these secondary but important clinical outcomes. Fourth, evidence regarding brief therapies other than CBT and PST was nonexistent or sparse. Finally, further research needs to expand participants beyond the mostly middle-aged, female, Caucasian subjects included in studies to date.

CONCLUSIONS

Based on our systematic review of two recent literature reviews and of seven additional RCTs, the collective evidence suggests that six to eight sessions of brief CBT or PST are more efficacious than control for the treatment of depression in primary care; however, the effects are modest (moderate strength of evidence). Current evidence suggests that these treatments might be effectively delivered by providers of various professional disciplines, provided they receive adequate training and supervision. This may be important in terms of balancing cost to the Veterans Health Administration with access to mental health treatment among Veterans. As the VA moves to the Patient-Aligned Care Team model of the patient-centered medical home, it is encouraging to find empirical evidence to support the provision of brief psychotherapy in primary care.

EVIDENCE REPORT

INTRODUCTION

Depressive disorders present a major public health concern. The prevalence of current depression among U.S. adults is 6.6%,[1] affecting up to 16 to 18% of the population over their lifetime.[2] High prevalence rates have also been noted in the Veteran population,[3] and particularly high rates have been found in primary care settings.[4] Although primary care physicians treat a high proportion of patients with depressive disorders,[5] the treatment of depression in primary care tends to be variable and suboptimal.[6] Because of this, it is a public health priority to identify treatments for depression that are effective, evidence-based, and suitable for dissemination in primary care.

The two evidence-based, first-line interventions for depression recommended by VA/Department of Defense (DoD) guidelines are pharmacotherapy and/or psychotherapy.[7] Based on several systematic reviews showing small-to-moderate benefit, the guideline recommends several classes of antidepressants as first-line therapy. Among psychotherapies, cognitive behavioral therapy (CBT), interpersonal psychotherapy (IPT) and problem-solving therapy (PST) are recommended as first-line treatment. For CBT and IPT, 16 to 20 sessions are recommended. Other psychotherapies are recommended for specific clinical situations, such as dialectical behavioral therapy (DBT), in combination with antidepressants for older adults with chronic major depressive disorder (MDD). In general, the evidence suggests that pharmacotherapy and psychotherapy are individually efficacious treatments and that there can be additive clinical benefit when these treatments are used in tandem.[8,9]

Despite persuasive evidence of effectiveness for both pharmacotherapy and psychotherapy in the treatment of depression, medication remains by far the most commonly utilized intervention in primary care settings.[10-12] However, there has been a growing interest in and commitment to the integration of psychotherapy and other mental health services into primary care settings,[13-15] perhaps most notably within the Veterans Health Administration.[16,17] Providing primary care patients with the option of receiving psychotherapy for their depression is an important objective for multiple reasons: there are many patients who, given the option, prefer psychotherapy to medication;[18-21] there is a need to provide alternative treatments for patients who do not improve on or cannot tolerate antidepressant medication;[22,23] and there may be unique benefits from psychotherapy in terms of costs[24-28] and relapse prevention.[29-31]

While there is good rationale for increasing the availability of psychological treatments for depression in primary care, there are also substantial barriers to incorporating psychotherapies into this setting. As with the prescription of antidepressant medication, there is a significant problem in delivering psychotherapy at the proper dose and with fidelity to the treatment model.[6,32] There are also a number of barriers to implementing psychotherapies in primary care that are distinct from barriers to providing effective pharmacological treatment. These barriers involve such pragmatic concerns as finding space in primary care clinics where psychotherapy can be provided in confidentiality and securing an adequate workforce with the proper training to meet the demand for psychotherapy.

Perhaps the most significant barrier to providing psychotherapies in primary care settings is that, unlike pharmacological treatment, many empirically supported psychotherapy treatment protocols consist of at least 12 to 16 weekly 1-hour sessions.[33,34] While this treatment duration is much abbreviated compared with older approaches to the provision of psychotherapy,[35] it is arguably still too intensive for reliable implementation in primary care settings.

Recognizing that time and resource constraints present important barriers to effectively implementing standard-duration psychotherapies (i.e., 12 to 20 sessions) for depression in primary care settings, this report evaluates whether psychotherapy for depression can be efficacious after a period of 8 or fewer sessions—what we define as brief psychotherapy. In examining the evidence on brief psychotherapies for depression, this report also aims to address issues of the amount of training necessary to deliver psychotherapeutic treatment effectively and the availability of data on key clinical outcomes like social functioning and satisfaction with treatment. Effectively treating depression in primary care patients is an important public health priority. With that in mind, this report endeavors to examine whether brief psychotherapies are often tailored specifically for primary care settings and are efficacious for the treatment of depression.

METHODS

TOPIC DEVELOPMENT

This review was commissioned by the Department of Veterans Affairs' Evidence-based Synthesis Program. The topic was selected after a formal topic nomination and prioritization process that included representatives from the Office of Mental Health Services, Health Services Research and Development, the Mental Health QUERI, and the Office of Mental Health and Primary Care Integration. The key research questions for this review were developed and refined after preliminary review of published peer-reviewed literature and consultation with VA and non-VA experts to select the patients and subgroups, interventions, outcomes, and settings addressed in this review.

The final key questions were as follows:

Key Question 1: For primary care patients with depressive disorders, are brief, evidence-based psychotherapies with durations of up to eight sessions more efficacious than control for depressive symptoms (i.e., on self-report and/or clinician-administered measures) and quality of life (i.e., functional status and/or health-related quality of life)?

Key Question 2: For primary care patients with depressive disorders treated with a brief, evidence-based psychotherapy, is there evidence that treatment effect may vary by the number of sessions delivered?

Key Question 3: For psychotherapies demonstrating clinically significant treatment effects, what are the characteristics of treatment providers (i.e., type of provider and training), and what are the modalities of therapy (i.e., individual/group, face-to-face/teletherapy/Internet-based)?

Key Question 4: How commonly reported are the key clinical outcomes of quality of life, social functioning, occupational status, patient satisfaction, and adverse treatment effects in randomized trials of psychotherapy?

We developed and followed a standard protocol for all steps of this review. Our approach was guided by the analytic framework shown in Figure 1.

Figure 1. Analytic Framework

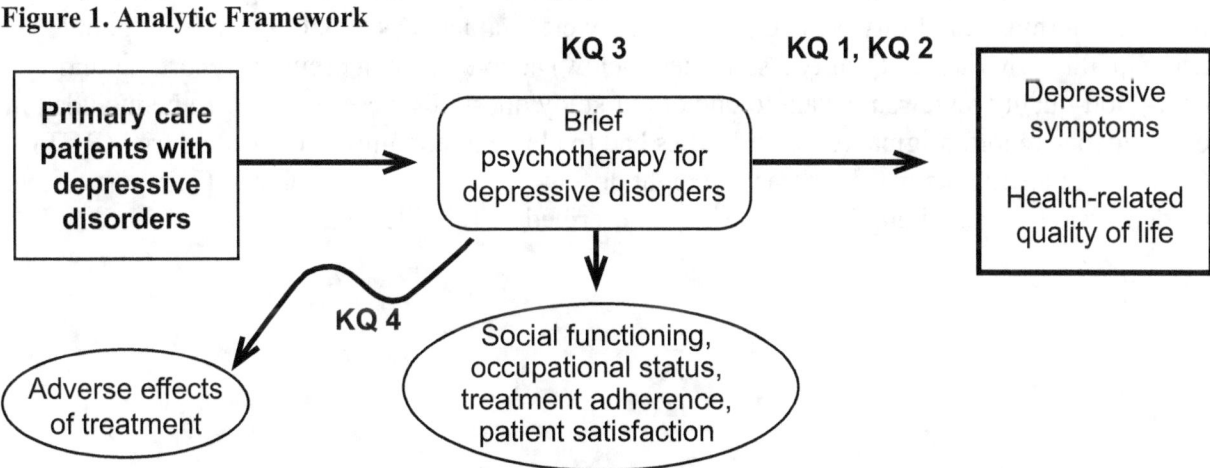

OVERALL APPROACH

We utilized a combined approach, identifying and evaluating existing, good-quality systematic reviews and supplementing these reviews by searching for and evaluating original research not included in these reviews. We were guided in this process by published recommendations for conducting "complex systematic reviews,"[36] which integrate findings from previous systematic reviews and findings from newly identified original research.

SEARCH STRATEGY

We conducted our search strategy using the following three complementary approaches:

1. We searched for relevant, good-quality, English-language systematic reviews in MEDLINE (via PubMed), Embase, and PsycINFO from database inception through May 2010.
2. We used a well-documented Internet-accessible database of 243 psychotherapy trials (www.psychotherapyrcts.org/index.php?id=3), current through January 2010, as a data source for original research. Using this database, we searched for studies coded as including adults with a mood disorder who received face-to-face psychotherapy at a dose of eight or fewer therapy sessions.
3. To identify any recent literature not yet catalogued in the Internet-accessible database, we searched for English-language publications in MEDLINE (via PubMed), Embase, and PsycINFO from January 2009 (one year prior to the search date of the online database) through August 1, 2010.

We developed search strategies in consultation with a master librarian. The search terms and MeSH headings for the search strategies appear in Appendix A. We supplemented electronic searching by examining the bibliographies of included studies and systematic review articles.

STUDY SELECTION

Using prespecified inclusion/exclusion criteria, two trained researchers reviewed the list of titles and abstracts, then selected articles, identified from any of the computerized and manual searches described above, for further review. Each article retrieved was reviewed using a brief screening form to determine eligibility. Systematic reviews were evaluated as "good," "fair," or "poor" using quality criteria (see Quality Assessment below) adapted from a previous report,[37,38] and only good-quality reviews relevant to one of our study questions were retained. To be included in our evidence report, original research studies had to (1) be a randomized controlled trial (RCT), (2) compare an eligible psychotherapy of eight or fewer sessions to control, and (3) report effects on depression. Detailed eligibility criteria are described in Table 1.

Table 1. Summary of Inclusion and Exclusion Criteria

Study characteristic	Inclusion criteria	Exclusion criteria
Study design	Randomized controlled trial	None
Population	Adults with major depressive disorder (MDD), dysthymic disorder, or subthreshold (minor) depression in acute-phase treatment	Treatment-resistant depression, postpartum depression, premenstrual dysphoric disorder, bipolar disorder, seasonal affective disorder, or double depression (i.e., MDD and dysthymia)
Interventions	Cognitive behavioral therapy (CBT) (including cognitive therapy and behavior therapy), interpersonal therapy (IPT), problem-solving therapy (PST), mindfulness-based cognitive therapy (MBCT), cognitive behavioral analysis system of psychotherapy (CBASP), dialectical behavioral therapy (DBT), functional analytic psychotherapy (FAP), acceptance and commitment therapy (ACT), or short-term psychodynamic therapy with ≤ 8 planned sessions	Generic counseling, life review therapy, psychoeducational therapy, supportive therapy, bibliotherapy, or Internet-based psychotherapies
Comparators	Waitlist, attention control, usual care Antidepressant medication if intervention is psychotherapy and an antidepressant	Another psychotherapy
Setting	Outpatient general medical or general mental health	Study conducted outside of North America, Western Europe, New Zealand, or Australia
Outcome	Depressive symptoms using a validated instrument reported at ≥ 6 weeks after randomization	None

DATA ABSTRACTION

For each newly identified primary research study, a trained researcher abstracted data from published reports into evidence tables (Appendix B). A second reviewer overread all data abstractions. We resolved disagreements by consensus among the first and second reviewer or by obtaining a third reviewer's opinion when consensus could not be reached. For eligible trials included in the two systematic reviews, we abstracted summary data from the reviews and supplemented these data by using the original publications when the reviews had incomplete information. We abstracted the following data: (1) study design and setting, (2) eligibility criteria, (3) exclusion criteria, (4) sample size, (5) demographics, (6) duration of followup, (7) depression clinical category, (8) intervention characteristics (e.g., type of therapy, mode, frequency, therapist), (9) comparator characteristics, (10) outcome measures, (11) results, and (12) adverse effects.

QUALITY ASSESSMENT

For systematic reviews, we assessed the comprehensiveness of the search strategy, the description and appropriateness of inclusion criteria, whether primary studies were assessed for quality and the adequacy of the quality measure, the reproducibility of methods to assess studies, whether the results of relevant studies were combined appropriately, whether heterogeneity and publication bias were assessed, and whether the conclusions were supported by the data presented. Systematic reviews were rated "good" if the conclusions were supported by the data presented and there were no important study limitations. For original research studies, we assessed risk of bias using the key quality criteria described in the Agency for Healthcare Research and Quality (AHRQ) *Methods Guide for Effectiveness and Comparative Effectiveness Reviews,*[39] adapted for this specific topic. We abstracted data on adequacy of randomization and allocation concealment, comparability of groups at baseline, blinding, completeness of followup and differential loss to followup, whether incomplete data were addressed appropriately, validity of outcome measures, and conflict of interest. Using these data elements, we assigned a summary quality score of "good," "fair," or "poor" to individual RCTs.

DATA SYNTHESIS

When good-quality systematic reviews were identified, we summarized the reviews' findings in narrative form. For original research studies that were not included in the systematic reviews, results were summarized descriptively in tables that include the study sample, intervention, comparator, duration of followup, and primary outcomes. We critically analyzed these studies to compare their characteristics, methods, and findings. We then evaluated whether the new evidence was likely to change estimates from prior reviews by considering the precision and stability of estimates from the original review, the number and size of the new studies relative to studies in the original review, the quality of the new studies, and the consistency in estimates and conclusions between the new evidence and the original reviews.[39] After considering these issues, we updated prior meta-analyses when substantial new evidence was available and a new summary estimate might lead to different conclusions.

Because studies did not use a single common instrument to measure depression severity, our meta-analysis used effect sizes to summarize intervention effects. Effect sizes were calculated for each study by subtracting (at posttest) the average score of the control group from the average score of the experimental group and dividing the result by the pooled standard deviations (SDs) of the experimental and control groups. A negative effect size indicates a greater effect in the intervention group. For example, an effect size of -0.5 indicates that the mean decline in depression severity for the experimental group is half an SD greater than the mean decline in the control group. We applied this convention of a negative effect size indicating a greater intervention effect to our summary of existing systematic reviews, converting signs when necessary for consistency. Effect sizes are commonly interpreted as small (0.2), moderate (0.5), and large (≥ 0.80).[40,41] To further aid interpretation of effect sizes, we converted these estimates to the number needed to treat (NNT) using the approach described by Kraemer.[41] When studies used more than one validated instrument to assess depression severity, we used the mean of the effect sizes so that each study (or control group) contributed only one effect size. When means and SDs were not reported, we used other statistics (e.g., event rates) to calculate the effect size. For studies with more than one active eligible intervention (e.g., behavioral therapy and cognitive therapy arms) compared to a single control, we combined the intervention arms to avoid lack of independence that would be created if we entered each intervention into the analysis separately.[42]

Because considerable heterogeneity was expected, we used a random effects model to calculate a pooled mean effect size. We used the Q statistic and the I^2 statistic to assess for heterogeneity in outcomes between studies. Because the Q statistic is underpowered, we consider a $p < 0.10$

as statistically significant. The I^2 statistic is an indicator of heterogeneity in percentages. The importance of between-study heterogeneity was represented by the I^2 statistic thresholds of 0% to 40% as likely not important, 30% to 60% as moderate, 50% to 90% as substantial, and 75% to 100% as considerable.[43] Publication bias was tested by inspecting the funnel plot of the meta-analysis. This procedure is based on the expectation that if no publication bias is present, the effect sizes will be dispersed equally on either side of the overall effect. However, this method has limited power to detect publication bias, particularly when the number of included studies is few.

We conducted preplanned subgroup analyses by study quality and type of control group. For other study characteristics (e.g., sessions delivered, type of depression), there was not sufficient variability and numbers of studies to conduct subgroup analyses. We used an influence analysis, recomputing the pooled mean effect by removing one study at a time, to determine the influence of individual studies on the overall effect. We used the computer program Comprehensive Meta-analysis, Version 2.2.021 (www.meta-analysis.com/pages/about_us.html), to conduct all meta-analyses.

Grading the Evidence for Each Key Question

We graded the strength of evidence for each key question using principles from the Grades of Recommendation, Assessment, Development, and Evaluation (GRADE) Working Group.[44] This approach assesses the strength of evidence for each critical outcome by considering risk of bias, consistency, directness, precision, and publication bias. Other domains relevant to observational designs were not pertinent to our review. After considering each domain, a summary rating of "high," "moderate," "low," or "insufficient" strength of evidence was assigned after discussion by two reviewers (Table 2).

Table 2. Definitions for Strength of Evidence Rating

Strength of evidence rating	Definition
High	Further research is very unlikely to change our confidence in the estimate of effect
Moderate	Further research is likely to have an important impact on our confidence in the estimate of effect and may change the estimate
Low	Further research is very likely to have an important impact on our confidence in the estimate of effect and is likely to change the estimate
Insufficient	Evidence on an outcome is absent or too weak, sparse, or inconsistent to estimate an effect

PEER REVIEW

A draft version of this report was sent to five peer reviewers. Their comments and our responses are presented in Appendix C.

RESULTS

Our general approach throughout the Results section is first to describe the relevant systematic reviews and then to describe the primary literature, with syntheses of the reviews and the primary literature occurring in conjunction with descriptions of the primary literature. This approach to integrating existing systematic reviews and new primary literature into a new "complex systematic review" was adopted and implemented in accordance with the recommendations for conducting complex systematic reviews proposed by Whitlock and colleagues.[36]

LITERATURE SEARCH AND STUDY CHARACTERISTICS

Systematic Reviews

Using the combined literature search of PubMed, Embase, PsycINFO, and Cochrane databases (Appendix A), we identified references for 560 potential systematic reviews (Figure 2). Of these, 528 were excluded at the title-and-abstract level, and 30 were excluded after conducting a full-text review. Two eligible reviews were retained: Cuijpers and colleagues[45] and Cape and colleagues.[46]

Cuijpers[45] completed a good-quality meta-analysis of 15 studies that examined psychotherapeutic interventions for depression in primary care. Studies were identified through an Internet-accessible database of psychotherapy trials[47] that was created by the authors via comprehensive literature searches in PubMed, PsycINFO, Embase, and the Cochrane Central Register of Controlled Trials from 1966 to December 2007. Included studies had interventions ranging in length from 6 to 16 sessions; only CBT and PST used 8 or fewer sessions. The majority of treatments were either CBT or PST, with two studies examining IPT and one study examining psychodynamic counseling. Most comparator conditions were care as usual (which was noted as being poorly described and variable in the reviewed studies), three were placebo, and two were waitlist. Half of the studies contained participants diagnosed with MDD, and the other half contained participants with other depressive conditions. Eight studies were conducted in the U.K., five in the U.S., and two in the Netherlands. The risk of bias varied across studies. Of the 15 trials, 13 assessed outcomes blind to treatment assignment, 10 were analyzed using the intent to treat principle, and dropout rates varied from 3.3 to 41.2%. The authors separated the seven studies with six or fewer sessions from the eight studies with more than six sessions; this subgroup analysis was of particular interest for the present review.

Brief Psychotherapy for Depression in Primary Care

Figure 2. Literature Flow Diagram

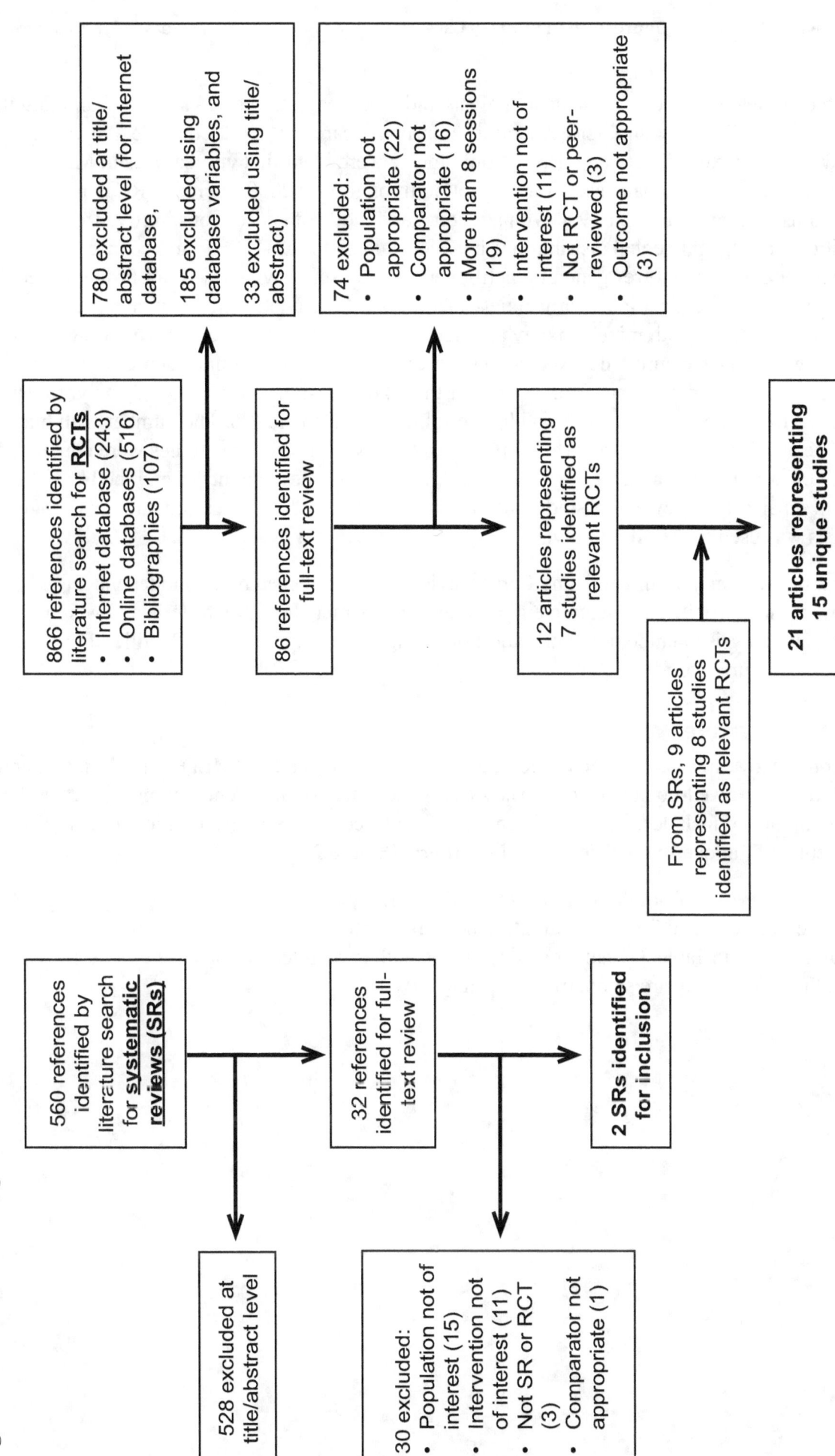

Cape[46] completed a good-quality meta-analysis and meta-regression of 34 studies examining the effectiveness of brief psychological therapies in primary care for anxiety disorders, depressive disorders, and mixed anxiety and depression. Studies were identified via searches in MEDLINE, Embase, and PsycINFO databases from inception through July 2008. Included RCTs had number of sessions ranging from 2.3 to 9.8, with a median and mode of six sessions. Active treatment conditions had roughly equal distributions between studies for CBT, PST, and counseling. All comparator conditions were "general practitioner care as usual," which was not further described. Seven studies included patients with anxiety disorders, 14 included patients with depression, and 13 included patients with mixed anxiety and depression. Of the 14 depression studies, 6 enrolled patients with MDD, 6 enrolled mixed depressive disorders including minor depression, and 2 enrolled only those with minor depression. For the 14 depression studies, 8 were analyzed using the intent-to-treat principle, and 10 had lost to followup less than 20%. The number with blinded outcome assessment was not reported. Approximately two-thirds of the studies were conducted in the U.K., with the remaining third conducted in other European countries and the U.S. The authors separately reviewed the studies of brief psychotherapy for depression, and this subgroup analysis was used in the present review.

After articles from the Cuijpers[45] and Cape[46] reviews were screened by two independent reviewers, nine articles representing eight unique studies met eligibility criteria and were retained for further analysis in tandem with the additional original research studies identified from the primary literature searches.

Primary Literature

The combined searches for primary literature in electronic databases (MEDLINE, Embase, and PsycINFO), in a well-documented Internet-accessible database of psychotherapy trials,[47] and in bibliographies of included studies (Appendix A) identified 866 citations. Of these, 12 articles representing 7 unique studies met eligibility criteria (Figure 2).

Study characteristics from the 15 relevant RCTs of brief psychotherapy—8 from the Cuijpers[45] and Cape[46] reviews and 7 from the additional RCTs identified in our primary literature search—are summarized in Table 3. Characteristics of psychotherapy interventions used in the 15 RCTs of brief psychotherapy are summarized in Table 4.

Table 3. Summary of Study Characteristics

	Author, year	Depressive disorder	Age mean (SD)	% Female	% White	Setting	Recruitment	Most distal followup[a]	Depression outcomes	Quality[b]
RCTs from systematic reviews	Barrett et al., 2001[48] and Frank et al., 2002[4]	Minor depression or dysthymia	43.6 (NR)	67%	89%	PC	Screening and referral	11 weeks	HRSD-17; HSCL-20	—
	Dowrick et al., 2000[5]	MDD, dysthymia, adjustment disorder, or other depression	NR; Range: 18-65	66%	NR	PC	Screening from census and registry	52 weeks	BDI	—
	Lynch et al., 1997[49]	Elevated depressive symptoms without MDD	48.4 (NR)	86%	NR	PC	Screening	7 weeks	HRSD; BDI	—
	Lynch et al., 2004[50]	Elevated depressive symptoms	38.5 (13.7)	83%	NR	PC	Screening	6 weeks	HRSD; BDI; DHP	—
	Mynors-Wallis et al., 1995[51]	MDD	37.1 (11.4)	77%	95%	PC	Referral	12 weeks	HRSD; BDI	—
	Scott et al., 1997[52]	MDD	41 (10.4)	67%	NR	PC	Referral	52 weeks	HRSD; BDI	Fair
	Ward et al., 2000[53] and King et al., 2000[54]	Depression or mixed anxiety depression	36.8 (12.2)	76%	89%	PC	Referral	52 weeks	BDI-21	Fair
	Williams et al., 2000[55] and Frank et al., 2002[4]	Dysthymia or minor depression	71 (7.1)	43%	76%	PC	Screening and referral	11 weeks	HSCL-D-20; HRSD	—
RCTs from primary literature searches	Barnhofer et al., 2009[56]	MDD or subthreshold MDD	41.9 (10.4)	68%	NR	MH	Advertisement and referral	8 weeks	BDI	Good
	Laidlaw et al., 2008[57]		74.0 (8.0)	73%	NR	PC	Referral	26 weeks	BDI; GDS; HRSD	Fair
	Mynors-Wallis et al., 2000[58]	MDD	34.5 (NR)	78%	93%	PC	Referral	52 weeks	HRSD; BDI	Good
	Nezu, 1986[59]	MDD	41.7 (12.8)	81%	NR	MH	Advertisement	26 weeks	BDI; MMPI-D	Fair
	Simon et al., 2004[60] and Simon et al., 2009[61]	Antidepressant and depressive symptoms	44.8 (15.5)	74%	80%	PC	Registry	24 weeks	SCL	Good
	Wilson, 1982[62]	Self-report of depression	38.8 (NR)	66%	NR	MH	Advertisement	26 weeks	BDI	Poor
	Wilson, 1983[63]	Self-report of depression	39.5 (NR)	80%	NR	MH	Advertisement	8 weeks	BDI; HRSD	Fair

[a] Weeks since baseline assessment.
[b] Quality assessments were conducted for the seven newly identified RCTs, and in order to conduct the meta-analysis on studies of brief CBT, quality assessments were completed for two studies that had been included in the systematic reviews.

Abbreviations: BDI = Beck Depression Inventory, DHP = Diabetes Health Profile, DIS = Diagnostic Interview Schedule, GDS = Geriatric Depression Scale, GP = general practitioner, HRSD = Hamilton Rating Scale for Depression, HSLC-D = Headache Specific Locus of Control-Depression, MDD = major depressive disorder, MH = mental health, MMPI-D = Minnesota Multiphasic Personality Inventory Depression Scale, MOS-D = Medical Outcomes Study-Depression, NR = not reported, PC = primary care, PRIME-MD = Primary Care Evaluation of Mental Disorders Patient Health Questionnaire, RDC = Research Diagnostic Criteria, SADS-L = Schedule for Affective Disorders and Schizophrenia–Lifetime Version, SCAN = Schedules for Clinical Assessment in Neuropsychiatry, SCL = Symptom Checklist

Table 4. Summary of Intervention Characteristics

	Author, year	Therapy	# sessions	Session length	Session frequency	Modality	Therapist	Treatment fidelity?	Therapy completed [n (%)]	Control
RCTs from systematic reviews	Barrett et al., 2001[48] and Frank et al., 2002[4]	PST (n = 80)	6	30 min	Ever 2 weeks	Individual	PhD psychologist	Yes	64 (80%)	Placebo (n = 81)
	Dowrick et al., 2000[5]	PST (n = 128)	6	30 min	NR	Individual	Psychologists, nurses, allied health professionals	Yes	80 (63%)	Waitlist (n = 189)
	Lynch et al., 1997[49]	PST (n = 15)	6	20 min	Weekly	Individual; telephone	Graduate students	No	11 (73%)	Usual care (n = 14)
	Lynch et al., 2004[50]	PST (n = 18)	6	NR	Weekly	Individual; telephone	Nurses	Yes	NR	Usual care (n = 18)
	Mynors-Wallis et al., 1995[51]	PST (n = 30)	6	30 min	Every 2 weeks	Individual	Experienced psychiatrist and trained GPs	No	28 (93%)	Placebo (n = 30)
	Scott et al., 1997[52]	CBT (n = 24)	6	30 min	Weekly	Individual	CBT therapist	Yes	18 (75%)	Usual care (n = 24)
	Ward et al., 2000[53] and King et al., 2000[54]	CBT (n = 63)	6	50 min	Weekly	Individual	Experienced psychologists	Yes	56 (89%)	Usual care (n = 67)
	Williams et al., 2000[55] and Frank et al., 2002[4]	PST (n = 138)	6	30 min	Every 2 weeks	Individual	PhD psychologist, social workers, master's-level counselors	Yes	108 (78%)	Medication; placebo (n = 140)
RCTs from primary literature searches	Barnhofer et al., 2009[56]	MBCT (n = 16)	8	2 hours	Weekly	Group	MBCT therapists	Yes	14 (88%)	TAU (n = 14)
	Laidlaw et al., 2008[57]	CBT (n = 21)	8	NR	NR	Individual	Master's-level psychologist	Yes	20 (95%)	TAU (n = 23)
	Mynors-Wallis et al., 2000[58]	PST + Med. (n = 35)	6	30 min	Every 2 weeks	Individual	Research practice nurse	No	34 (97%)	Medication alone (n = 36)
	Nezu, 1986[59]	PST (n = 12)	8	1.75 hours	Weekly	Group	Graduate students	Yes	11 (92%)	Waitlist control (n = 9)
	Simon et al., 2004[60] and Simon et al., 2009[61]	CBT+TCM (n = 195)	8	35 min	Every ≈1.5 weeks[a]	Individual; Telephone	Master's-level psychologist	No	167 (86%)	TCM (n = 207)
	Wilson, 1982[62]	CBT (n ≈ 32)[b]	7	1 hour	Weekly	Individual	Graduate students	NR	21 (66%)	Minimal contact[c] (n ≈ 32)[b]
	Wilson, 1983[63]	CBT (n = 16)	8	1 hour	Weekly	Individual	NR	No	12 (75%)	Waitlist (n = 9)

[a] Weekly sessions for first 4 weeks, with frequency ranging from every 1 to 4 weeks for remaining four sessions.
[b] Estimate based on data provided in article.
[c] Minimal contact consisted of two 1-hour nondirective therapy sessions to coincide with medication refills.

Abbreviations: CBT = cognitive behavioral therapy (includes cognitive therapy and behavioral therapy), MBCT = mindfulness-based cognitive therapy, min = minutes, NR = not reported, PST = problem-solving therapy, TAU = treatment as usual, TCM = telephone case management

Of the 15 unique studies, 6 studies were conducted in the U.S., 6 in the U.K., 2 in Australia, and 1 recruited patients across several European countries. All studies were conducted with English-speaking patients. Patients were predominantly treated in primary care, with 11 trials taking place in a primary care setting, and 4 taking place in a mental health outpatient setting. Recruitment strategies varied such that participants were recruited via screening in five studies, referral from a provider in eight studies, advertisement in four studies, and registries in two studies; many trials used more than one recruitment method. Studies had varying diagnostic criteria for inclusion, with six trials specifically allowing for the inclusion of subthreshold depression (e.g., minor depression, adjustment disorder, depressive symptoms), five requiring a diagnosis of MDD, and the remaining four using other criteria (e.g., beginning antidepressant, self-report of depression).

The intervention in eight studies was PST; in six studies, CBT; and in one study, mindfulness-based cognitive therapy (MBCT). No trials of other psychotherapies using interventions of eight sessions or fewer were identified. Interventions were monitored for treatment fidelity in nine studies. Included studies most commonly measured depressive symptoms using the clinician-administered Hamilton Rating Scale for Depression (HRSD) and the self-report Beck Depression Inventory (BDI); only one study used neither of these measures. Even though no study extended treatment beyond eight sessions, followup duration was less than 6 months for seven studies and was 6 months or greater for eight studies. In all but one study, females outnumbered males by a ratio of at least 2 to 1. The average age for study participants ranged from 35 to 48 years of age in 13 of the 15 studies, with the 2 remaining studies having participants with average ages of 71 and 74 years of age. These two studies of elderly patients had mixed results: one found small to no benefit in elderly patients receiving PST for depression,[55] and the other found significant and sustained benefit in elderly patients receiving CBT for depression.[57] Most studies did not report race, and the six studies that did report race had heavily Caucasian samples. Only two study samples included any Veteran representation.[48,55] In both samples, Veterans composed only a portion of the overall sample, and data on Veterans were not presented separately.

Quality assessments were conducted for the seven RCTs identified in the primary literature searches—one was rated as poor, three as fair, and three as good. Fair and poor studies were often rated as such due to inadequately addressing incomplete outcome data and not having outcome assessors who were blind to treatment assignment. In order to conduct the meta-analysis on studies of brief CBT, quality assessments were completed for two studies that had been included in the systematic reviews; both were rated as fair.

KEY QUESTION 1. For primary care patients with depressive disorders, are brief, evidence-based psychotherapies with durations of up to eight sessions more efficacious than control for depressive symptoms (i.e., on self-report and/or clinician-administered measures) and quality of life (i.e., functional status and/or health-related quality of life)?

Systematic Reviews

Cuijpers'[45] systematic review of 15 RCTs found psychological treatment from a range of 6 to 16 sessions to be significantly more effective than control for treatment of depression in primary care (ES -0.31, 95% CI -0.45 to -0.17, NNT = 5.75). They found significantly larger effect sizes for studies in which participants were referred by their general practitioner (GP) (ES -0.43, 95% CI -0.58 to -0.28, NNT = 4.20) than for studies in which participants were recruited through systematic screening (ES -0.13, 95% CI -0.34 to 0.08, NNT – 13.51). The lower effect size for brief psychotherapy in the subgroup of primary care patients recruited through systematic screening was suggested as the reason why an initial comparison favored brief psychotherapy delivered in non–primary care settings (ES -0.67, 95% CI -0.75 to -0.58, NNT = 2.75) compared to brief psychotherapy delivered in primary care settings (ES -0.31, 95% CI -0.45 to -0.17, NNT = 5.75). The authors found no significant difference between studies in which participants were diagnosed with MDD (ES -0.21, 95% CI -0.42 to 0.00, NNT = 8.47) and studies in which participants' depressive symptomatology was alternatively determined (ES -0.40, 95% CI -0.56 to -0.23, NNT = 4.50). The multiple subgroup analyses conducted in this good-quality review allowed for the authors to present both robust and nuanced findings. In regard to psychotherapies with a fewer number of sessions, the authors found that, compared to control, psychotherapies of ≤ 6 sessions (n = 7) had a small but significant positive effect for the treatment of depression in primary care (ES -0.25, 95% CI -0.48 to -0.02, NNT = 7.14). HRQOL outcomes were not reported in this review.

Cape's[46] meta-analysis of 34 studies examined efficacy in regard to treatment type and in regard to three diagnostic categories: anxiety, depression, and mixed depression and anxiety. For certain analyses, they combined patients with diagnoses in the latter two categories. They found smaller treatment effects when CBT was used for mixed depression and anxiety (ES -0.26, 95% CI -0.44 to -0.08) than for anxiety (i.e., predominantly panic disorder and generalized anxiety disorder; ES -1.06, 95% CI -1.31 to -0.80). They found similar small effect sizes for PST for depression and mixed depression and anxiety (ES -0.21, 95% CI -0.37 to -0.05) and for counseling for depression and mixed depression and anxiety (ES -0.32, 95% CI -0.52 to -0.11). The examination of different psychotherapies in three different diagnostic groups (i.e., depression, anxiety, and mixed depression and anxiety) was a particular strength of this review. In regard to brief psychotherapies specifically for patients with depression, the authors found a significant but small effect favoring brief CBT over usual GP care for depression (ES -0.33, 95% CI -0.60 to -0.06) and found a positive but statistically nonsignificant effect for PST over usual GP care (ES -0.26, 95% CI -0.49 to 0.03). No significant differences in efficacy were found between CBT and PST. HRQOL outcomes were not reported in this review.

Primary Literature

Among the seven studies that we discovered were not included in the systematic reviews were two studies of PST, one of MBCT, and four of CBT. The 4 studies of CBT randomized 535 participants to treatment or control, whereas the 2 relevant studies of brief CBT covered in the systematic reviews randomized 178 participants to treatment or control. Because of the number of CBT trials not considered in the previous 2 systematic reviews, we conducted a meta-analysis of the 6 trials involving 713 patients to evaluate the effects of brief CBT (6 to 8 sessions) for depression.

For the 6 trials, study quality was rated as good (n = 1), fair (n = 4), or poor (n = 1). Studies enrolled patients with MDD (n = 2), depressive symptoms (n = 2), depression or mixed anxiety depression (n = 1), or patients with depressive symptoms who were starting an antidepressant (n = 1). Control conditions were treatment as usual in four of the six trials, and in two trials control conditions contained an additional therapeutic component beyond usual care.[60,62] Care as usual in these trials was typically described as allowing the primary care provider their usual discretion in treating depression; some studies noted that this could include antidepressant medication, counseling, or referral, whereas other studies did not specify the range of options left open to providers.

Participants receiving brief CBT for depression were more likely than participants receiving a control treatment to have reduced symptoms of depression (ES -0.42, 95% CI -0.74 to -0.10), but treatment effects differed significantly across studies (Cochran Q = 13.74, p = 0.03, I^2 = 56%) (Figure 3). The ES of -0.42 corresponds to an NNT of approximately 4.5. A funnel plot did not suggest significant publication bias, but with only six studies, this method has limited power to detect publication bias. To examine the moderate level of variability present, we conducted an influence analysis. In this analysis, the summary estimate ranged from -0.24 to -0.53, with the trial by Wilson[63] having the greatest influence. This trial was the only one of the six CBT studies to use a waitlist control condition as the comparator. Based on a priori hypotheses of variables that might influence the effect size estimate, we conducted two sensitivity analyses: in the first, we removed poor-quality studies from the meta-analysis; in the second, we removed both poor-quality studies and studies that used nontherapeutic comparator conditions (e.g., waitlist) from the meta-analysis. In the meta-analysis with the poor-quality study removed,[62] brief CBT for depression continued to be significantly more effective than control (ES -0.50, 95% CI -0.91 to -0.09), but treatment effects remained significantly heterogeneous (Cochran Q = 13.71, p = 0.008, I^2 = 71%). With the poor-quality study[62] and the study with a waitlist comparator[63] removed, treatment effects of brief CBT for depression were smaller (ES -0.24, 95% CI -0.42 to -0.06) but homogeneous (Cochran Q = 1.44, p = 0.70, I^2 = 0%). This effect size corresponds to an NNT of approximately eight. These results are highly consistent with both Cuijpers'[45] and Cape's[46] estimates of effect size for brief CBT for the treatment of depression.

Figure 3. Meta-analysis of Brief CBT for Depression

Study Name	Outcome	Std diff in means	Standard error	p-Value	Std diff in means and 95% CI	Relative weight
Wilson 1982a	Self-report	-0.25	0.44	0.57		9.34
Wilson 1982b	Self-report	-0.23	0.43	0.59		9.73
Wilson 1983	Combined	-2.13	0.53	0.00		7.15
Scott 1997	Combined	-0.48	0.35	0.16		12.63
King 2000	Self-report	-0.34	0.19	0.06		21.47
Simon 2004	Self-report	-0.16	0.12	0.18		25.73
Laidlaw 2008	Combined	-0.36	0.32	0.26		13.94
		-0.42	0.16	0.01		

-1.00   -0.50   0.00   0.50   1.00

Favors CBT   Favors Control

Meta Analysis

The 2 studies of PST identified in the primary literature searches and not included in the systematic reviews randomized 92 participants to treatment or control, whereas the 6 studies of PST covered in the systematic reviews randomized 881 participants. Thus, we did not conduct an updated meta-analysis for PST. The two studies of PST identified in the primary literature searches were conducted by Mynors-Wallis and colleagues[58] and Nezu.[59] In a good-quality trial involving 71 participants, Mynors-Wallis[58] found that adding six sessions of PST to antidepressant medication did not significantly enhance outcomes over treatment with antidepressant medication alone after 12 weeks (60% recovered versus 67%). They also found that after 12 and 52 weeks antidepressant alone was not significantly different in effectiveness from PST alone. In a small, fair-quality trial, Nezu[59] found eight sessions of PST to be significantly more effective in reducing depressive symptoms than either problem-focused therapy or a waitlist control at 8 weeks (t = 3.25, p < .01). These results are consistent with both Cape's[46] and Cuijpers'[45] conclusion that PST is an efficacious option for the treatment of depression.

No studies of MBCT were included in the systematic reviews. We identified a single good-quality study of MBCT that met our inclusion criteria.[56] This study randomized 30 subjects with MDD or subthreshold depression, recruited from a mental health setting, and found 8 sessions of MBCT to be more efficacious than treatment as usual at reducing depressive symptoms at 8 weeks (F = 13.42, p = 0.001).

Quality of life was too infrequently reported across studies to synthesize into any quantitative analyses. The two studies of CBT from the present meta-analysis that included data on quality of life did not find significant differences on quality-of-life outcomes between participants in the CBT conditions compared to participants in the control conditions.[53,57] No other trials from the studies identified via the primary literature searches included data on quality of life. The frequency with which data on quality of life were reported is considered in Key Question 4.

KEY QUESTION 2. For primary care patients with depressive disorders treated with a brief, evidence-based psychotherapy, is there evidence that treatment effect may vary by the number of sessions delivered?

Cuijpers[45] found a small difference in effect size between psychotherapies of six or fewer sessions (ES -0.25, 95% CI -0.48 to -0.02) compared to psychotherapies of seven or more sessions (ES -0.36, 95% CI -0.54 to -0.17), but confidence intervals overlapped. Should a more adequately powered meta-analysis be possible in the future, the means and confidence intervals surrounding these effect sizes leave room for the possibility of a clinically significant difference between brief and standard-duration psychotherapies.

Cape[46] did not conduct a comparison based on number of psychotherapy sessions delivered, as their review was limited to therapies of fewer than 10 sessions in duration. Similarly, because the present review included only studies with eight or fewer sessions and there was little variability in session number (six to eight), an analysis of whether treatment effect varies by quantity of therapy sessions could not be conducted.

KEY QUESTION 3. For psychotherapies demonstrating clinically significant treatment effects, what are the characteristics of treatment providers (i.e., type of provider and training), and what are the modalities of therapy (i.e., individual/group, face-to-face/teletherapy/Internet-based)?

Of the 15 RCTs evaluating brief therapies, 13 used an individual psychotherapy format, and 2 relied on a group therapy format. Two of the individual PST treatments and one of the individual CBT treatments were conducted over the phone. PST treatment providers included psychologists in three studies, nurses in three studies, graduate students in two studies, and other health professionals in three studies (e.g., GPs, allied health professionals, social workers). CBT treatment providers included psychologists in three studies, graduate students in one study, and nonidentified professionals in two studies. The MBCT treatment provider had completed an internship under the supervision of an expert MBCT therapist. There was substantial variability in the level of detail provided about therapists' training. Most therapists were noted either as having previous experience in the intervention treatment model or as having been trained and supervised for study purposes by one of the study's investigators.

While the number of sessions ranged only from six to eight, there was substantial variance in the intensity at which psychotherapies were provided. The most intensive therapy, MBCT, required 2 hours per week for 8 weeks, whereas multiple PST protocols required only 30-minute sessions spaced approximately every other week. Although it would appear that the two were separated by a difference of only two sessions, the intensity was different because the MBCT protocol specified a total of 16 hours of treatment, whereas the PST protocols specified a total of only 3.5 hours (first session is typically 1 hour). Three of the CBT protocols consisted of 50- to 60-minute sessions, and two consisted of 30- to 35-minute sessions.

Quantitative syntheses to examine differences on the basis of treatment intensity, provider type, individual versus group, and telephone versus in-person could not be completed because there was not an adequate number of studies in each of these subgroups.

KEY QUESTION 4. How commonly reported are the key clinical outcomes of quality of life, social functioning, occupational status, patient satisfaction, and adverse treatment effects in randomized trials of psychotherapy?

Neither of the two systematic reviews reported on quality of life, social functioning, occupational status, patient satisfaction, or adverse treatment effects. Of the 15 RCTs contained in this evidence report, 5 reported HRQOL, 5 reported social functioning, 0 reported occupational status, 2 reported patient satisfaction with treatment, and 1 reported adverse treatment effects (Table 5). The most commonly used measure of quality of life for studies that examined this clinical outcome was the SF-36. The one study that reported adverse treatment effects examined the side effects of taking psychotropic medication in tandem with psychotherapy.

Table 5. Key Clinical Outcome Measures

	Study	Quality of life	Social functioning	Occupational status	Patient satisfaction	Adverse treatment effects
RCTs from systematic reviews	Barrett et al, 2001[48] and Frank et al., 2002[4]	Yes, SF-36	NR	NR	NR	NR
	Dowrick et al., 2000[5]	Yes, SF-36	NR	NR	NR	NR
	Lynch et al., 1997[49]	NR	Yes	NR	NR	NR
	Lynch et al., 2004[50]	NR	NR	NR	NR	NR
	Mynors-Wallis et al., 1995[51]	NR	Yes	NR	Yes	NR
	Scott et al., 1997[52]	NR	NR	NR	NR	NR
	Ward et al., 2000[53] and King et al., 2000[54]	Yes, EuroQoL	Yes	NR	NR	NR
	Williams et al., 2000[55] and Frank et al., 2002[4]	Yes, SF-36	NR	NR	NR	NR
RCTs from primary literature searches	Barnhofer et al., 2009[56]	NR	NR	NR	NR	NR
	Laidlaw et al., 2008[57]	Yes, WHOQOL-BREF	Yes, social relationships	NR	NR	NR
	Mynors-Wallis et al., 2000[58]	NR	Yes, Social Adjustment Scale	NR	NR	Yes, medication side effects
	Nezu, 1986[59]	NR	NR	NR	NR	NR
	Simon et al., 2004[60] and Simon et al., 2009[61]	NR	NR	NR	Yes	NR
	Wilson, 1982[62]	NR	NR	NR	NR	NR
	Wilson, 1983[63]	NR	NR	NR	NR	NR

Abbreviations: NR = not reported, WHOQOL = World Health Organization Quality of Life

DISCUSSION

Based on our complex systematic review of two recent literature reviews and seven additional RCTs not considered in these previous reviews, the collective evidence suggests that six to eight sessions of brief CBT or PST for acute-phase treatment in primary care are more efficacious than usual care, but effects are modest. However, insofar as usual care consists of treatments that are intended to be effective and that may in some cases be "best practice" treatments, usual care could represent a more potent control condition than placebo controls used in antidepressant trials. Also, there is some evidence to indicate that brief psychotherapy may be more efficacious when patients are referred at the discretion of their primary care provider than when patients are selected for treatment on the basis of systematic depression screening. We conclude that brief psychotherapy may prove an efficacious treatment option for a number of patients with depression in VA primary care settings. Because the reviewed studies contained little Veteran representation, relied heavily on samples of predominantly middle-aged Caucasian females, and frequently excluded patients with complex or comorbid psychiatric conditions, additional research is needed to more definitively confirm the effectiveness of brief psychotherapy for depression in the Veteran population (Key Question 1).

Whether brief psychotherapies significantly differ in efficacy from standard-duration psychotherapies (12 to 20 sessions) is a question that we could not directly address given the limited range of session duration (6 to 8) in the 15 studies included in this review. Cuijpers' (2009) review[45] found no statistically significant differences between psychotherapies delivered in six or fewer sessions compared to psychotherapies delivered over seven or more sessions; however, the wide confidence intervals for effect sizes of brief and standard-duration psychotherapies leave open the possibility of clinically significant differences (Key Question 2).

Our review found that brief psychotherapies have been provided by an array of trained health care professionals, including non–mental health professionals. The efficacious treatments included in this review were provided not only by psychologists but also by graduate students, nurses, general practitioners, and other allied health professionals who had received training and supervision specific to the intervention being conducted. Details about training were sparse, meaning that the degree of training necessary to replicate studies' results is uncertain (Key Question 3). Finally, we discovered that effects on occupational status, patient satisfaction with treatment, and adverse treatment effects were seldom reported; HRQOL and social functioning were more commonly reported but still only considered in less than half the trials examined in this review (Key Question 4).

Depressive disorders cause enormous human suffering and impose a high economic burden. Ensuring access to evidence-based treatments for Veterans is critical to the VA mission. The current emphasis on evidence-based care management in the VA has the potential to significantly enhance the usual care of depression in VA primary care settings, and the Primary Care/Mental Health Integration program in the VA represents an important organizational strategy to improve access and the quality of mental health care. If the VA were to expand its capability to provide brief psychotherapy for primary care patients in the acute phase of depression, this too has the potential to improve access and quality. Fewer sessions would mean that the same workforce could provide treatment to a larger number of patients, potentially more cost-effectively. In addition, clinicians from a variety of disciplines, if given adequate training and under appropriate supervision, may be able to provide brief therapies, further expanding access. Although the exact training was often incompletely described, many studies used focused training with non–mental health specialists, followed by fidelity monitoring to ensure quality. Fidelity monitoring may be a key component of replicating the positive treatment effects, particularly with generalist clinicians. Within the VA, a range of providers could be considered, including nurses, nurse practitioners, primary care physicians, social workers, and chaplains. However, given the current nursing shortage and high demands on primary care physicians, any change or expansion in roles would need to be considered carefully.

If non–mental health professionals were to assume the role of providing brief therapies, patients should be screened carefully for those without high complexity, and oversight should be provided by qualified mental health professionals to ensure the safety of the patient. In the VA, integrated primary care/mental health teams often consist of primary care clinicians, psychiatrists, psychologists, and nurses and may provide an ideal context and support system in which to implement such a model.

One of our key questions was to assess how frequently key clinical outcomes were assessed. Review results revealed a striking lack of consistency in assessing and reporting important outcome measures. Of the 15 RCTs contained in this review, only 5 reported HRQOL, 5 reported social functioning, 0 reported of occupational status, 2 reported patient satisfaction with treatment, and 1 reported adverse treatment effects. Evaluating the efficacy of treatment is clearly important; however, without measuring key clinical outcomes like quality of life, social functioning, and occupational functioning, we constrict ourselves to understanding only a very limited range of how psychotherapies can impact mental and physical health.

STRENGTHS AND LIMITATIONS

Our study has a number of strengths, including a protocol-driven review, a comprehensive search, careful quality assessment, and rigorous quantitative synthesis methods. For the included systematic reviews, we verified outcomes reported and supplemented the descriptions of included trials by abstracting missing data from the primary publications. We also combined a narrative review of recent, good-quality systematic reviews with new meta-analyses when indicated. This approach allowed us to capitalize on the strengths and often detailed analyses performed in existing reviews while updating those results to include the most recent and relevant studies.

However, several questions still remain. First, the efficacy of brief psychotherapy modalities other than CBT and PST could not be determined. Although we had hoped to review a variety of interventions, CBT and PST were the only treatments in our review for which more than one trial had been completed. Second, it is not clear if efficacy differs by the number of treatment sessions. This was a key question for our review that we were unable to answer. For CBT and PST, six to eight sessions has a small, beneficial effect compared to usual care, but a lower bound or dose-response relationship could not be determined. Third, the studies included in this review were composed primarily of Caucasian, middle-aged females. This limits applicability to the VA and to many other segments of society. Research is needed to evaluate whether results are applicable across diverse populations. Fourth, it remains unclear whether the efficacy of brief psychotherapies varies according to depression severity (i.e., mild, moderate, severe). Fifth, major intervention outcomes (e.g., quality of life, social functioning, occupational status) are measured too infrequently. While these outcomes are often considered "secondary," they are critical in evaluating the safety and generalizability of treatments for real-world practice.

Despite these limitations, it appears that brief psychotherapy is effective in primary care settings in the acute-phase treatment of depression. Increasing the availability of psychotherapy, either through enlarging the pool of mental health professionals or by training non–mental health professionals, will advance the VA toward its mission of providing easy access to care for Veterans.[64]

CONCLUSIONS

We identified two systematic reviews and 15 trials of brief psychotherapy (i.e., ≤ 8 sessions) for depression, encompassing 1716 patients with MDD or depressive symptomatology. Both systematic reviews concluded that brief CBT and PST are efficacious for the acute-phase treatment of depression in primary care. This conclusion was corroborated by our analyses that included seven additional studies. Table 6 summarizes the strength of evidence for the question of whether brief psychotherapies are more efficacious than control for depressive symptoms. GRADE criteria were not applicable to the other key questions.

Table 6. Summary of the Strength of Evidence for Key Question 1

Number of studies (subjects)	Domains pertaining to strength of evidence				Magnitude of effect and strength of evidence
	Risk of Bias: Design/Quality	Consistency	Directness	Precision	Standardized mean difference (95% CI)
Key Question 1: Efficacy of brief psychotherapies					
Brief CBT 6 (713)	RCTs/Fair	Consistent	Direct	Some imprecision	-0.42 (-0.10 to -0.74) Moderate
Brief PST 8 (973)	RCTs/Good	Consistent	Direct	Some imprecision	-0.26 (-0.49 to -0.30) Moderate
MBCT 1 (30)	RCT/Good	NA	Direct	Serious imprecision	Low
Other therapies	NA	NA	NA	NA	Insufficient

FUTURE RESEARCH

The present review confirmed that brief psychotherapies (i.e., ≤ 8 sessions), such as brief CBT and brief PST, are efficacious as acute-phase treatments for depression. However, many questions remain to be answered about the effectiveness of brief psychotherapy. First, future research should rigorously test whether brief psychotherapies are of comparable efficacy to standard-duration psychotherapies (i.e., 12 to 20 sessions). This question was not directly tested by any trials in our review. Hence, our analysis of this question relied on pooled comparisons of various treatment durations from different trials, a method that is vulnerable to multiple confounders. Future research should include RCTs that compare psychotherapies that differ according to the number of sessions.

Existing research has also been limited by an inadequate consideration of patient outcomes. Accordingly, we advise future researchers to assess longer term outcomes after the conclusion of brief psychotherapies (e.g., 6 months or longer). Researchers should also assess a broader set of outcomes, such as social functioning, occupational status, and quality of life, instead of solely assessing depression severity. Quality-of-life measures are especially desirable as these allow for the computation of cost-effectiveness and cost-utility ratios, which are crucial for informing policy decisions.

Another priority for future research should be to evaluate whether the administration of brief psychotherapies in primary care settings actually produces the benefits that proponents claim. These include claims that (1) brief psychotherapies provided in the primary care context reduce the stigma of receiving treatment for mental health problems, (2) providing brief psychotherapies broadens the population that will initiate and complete treatment by placing a lower time burden on patients, and (3) brief psychotherapies increase the cost-effectiveness of psychotherapy. Proponents have also claimed that brief psychotherapies can be used to prevent the development of MDD in at-risk patients, such as patients with minor depression. These hypotheses should be tested empirically.

Finally, it is crucial to assess which types of brief psychotherapies can be provided with high treatment fidelity and efficacy and by which types of providers. Additional studies are needed to determine whether brief psychotherapies other than CBT and PST are efficacious. Also, an important consideration to be assessed is patient preferences for different treatment modalities and providers. Further, more research is needed to determine which providers are best suited to provide brief therapies. In the VA, these providers could include not only mental health professionals like psychologists, psychiatrists, and social workers but also appropriately trained and supervised registered nurses, nurse practitioners, physician's assistants, primary care physicians, and chaplains.

The VA has been a leader in fostering models of integrated primary care and mental health care, and in doing so, the VA is in a unique position to address many of the previously stated research needs within the context of integrated health care teams.

REFERENCES

1.   Current depression among adults---United States, 2006 and 2008. MMWR Morb Mortal Wkly Rep 2010;59(38):1229-35.

2.   Kessler RC, Berglund P, Demler O, et al. The epidemiology of major depressive disorder: results from the National Comorbidity Survey Replication (NCS-R). JAMA 2003;289(23):3095-105.

3.   Hankin CS, Spiro A, 3rd, Miller DR, et al. Mental disorders and mental health treatment among U.S. Department of Veterans Affairs outpatients: the Veterans Health Study. Am J Psychiatry 1999;156(12):1924-30.

4.   Frank E, Rucci P, Katon W, et al. Correlates of remission in primary care patients treated for minor depression. Gen Hosp Psychiatry 2002;24(1):12-9.

5.   Dowrick C, Dunn G, Ayuso-Mateos JL, et al. Problem solving treatment and group psychoeducation for depression: multicentre randomised controlled trial. Outcomes of Depression International Network (ODIN) Group. BMJ 2000;321(7274):1450-4.

6.   Wang PS, Lane M, Olfson M, et al. Twelve-month use of Mental Health Services in the United States - Results from the National Comorbidity Survey Replication. Arch Gen Psychiatry 2005;62(6):629-640.

7.   The Management of MDD Working Group: VA/DoD Clinical Practice Guideline for Management of Major Depressive Disorder (MDD). Washington, DC: Department of Veterans Affairs and Department of Defense, 2009. Available at: www.healthquality. va.gov/mdd/mdd_full09_c.pdf. Accessed January 12, 2011.

8.   Oestergaard S, Moldrup C. Optimal duration of combined psychotherapy and pharmacotherapy for patients with moderate and severe depression: A meta-analysis. J Affect Disord 2010.

9.   Pampallona S, Bollini P, Tibaldi G, et al. Combined pharmacotherapy and psychological treatment for depression: a systematic review. Arch Gen Psychiatry 2004;61(7):714-9.

10.   Katon W, Robinson P, Von Korff M, et al. A multifaceted intervention to improve treatment of depression in primary care. Arch Gen Psychiatry 1996;53(10):924-32.

11.   Gill D, Hatcher S. Antidepressants for depression in medical illness. Cochrane Database of Systematic Reviews 2000, Issue 4. Art. No.: CD001312.

12.   Schulberg HC, Block MR, Madonia MJ, et al. The 'usual care' of major depression in primary care practice. Arch Fam Med 1997;6(4):334-9.

13.   Haas LJ. *Handbook of primary care psychology.* Oxford; New York: Oxford University Press; 2004.

14.   DeLeon PH, N.P. R, Smedley BD. The future is primary care. In: Frank RG, McDaniel SH, Bray JH, Heldring M, eds. Primary care psychology. Washington: American Psychological Association; 2004:317-325.

15.   Cummings NA. A history of behavioral healthcare: A perspective from a lifetime of involvement. In: Cummings NA, O'Donohue W, Hayes SC, Follette V, eds. Integrated behavioral healthcare: Positioning mental health practice with medical/surgical practice. San Diego: Academic Press; 2001:1-18.

16.   Zeiss AM, Karlin BE. Integrating mental health and primary care services in the Department of Veterans Affairs health care system. J Clin Psychol Med Settings 2008;15(1):73-8.

17.   Post EP, Van Stone WW. Veterans Health Administration primary care-mental health integration initiative. N C Med J 2008;69(1):49-52.

18.   Backenstrass M, Joest K, Frank A, et al. Preferences for treatment in primary care: a comparison of nondepressive, subsyndromal and major depressive patients. Gen Hosp Psychiatry 2006;28(2):178-80.

19.   Chilvers C, Dewey M, Fielding K, et al. Antidepressant drugs and generic counselling for treatment of major depression in primary care: randomised trial with patient preference arms. BMJ 2001;322(7289):772-5.

20.   Raue P, Schulberg HC. Psychotherapy and patient preferences for the treatment of major depression in primary care. In: Henri MJ, ed. Trends in depression research. Hauppauge, NY: Nova Science Publishers; 2007:31-51.

21.   van Schaik DJF, Klijn AFJ, van Hout HPJ, et al. Patients' preferences in the treatment of depressive disorder in primary care. Gen Hosp Psychiatry 2004;26(3):184-189.

22.   Trivedi RB, Nieuwsma JA, Williams JW, Jr., et al. Evidence synthesis for determining the efficacy of psychotherapy for treatment resistant depression. Washington, DC: Department of Veterans Affairs; October 2009. Available at: www.hsrd.research.va.gov/publications/esp/Depression-Q3.pdf. Accessed January 12, 2011.

23.   Thase ME, Friedman ES, Biggs MM, et al. Cognitive therapy versus medication in augmentation and switch strategies as second-step treatments: a STAR*D report. Am J Psychiatry 2007;164(5):739-52.

24.   Lave JR, Frank RG, Schulberg HC, et al. Cost-effectiveness of treatments for major depression in primary care practice. Arch Gen Psychiatry 1998;55(7):645-51.

25.   Schoenbaum M, Unutzer J, Sherbourne C, et al. Cost-effectiveness of practice-initiated quality improvement for depression: results of a randomized controlled trial. JAMA 2001;286(11):1325-30.

26.   Schulberg HC, Raue PJ, Rollman BL. The effectiveness of psychotherapy in treating depressive disorders in primary care practice: clinical and cost perspectives. Gen Hosp Psychiatry 2002;24(4):203-12.

27.   Antonuccio DO, Thomas M, Danton WG. A cost-effectiveness analysis of cognitive behavior therapy and fluoxetine (prozac) in the treatment of depression. Behavior Therapy 1997;28(2):187-210.

28.   Vos T, Corry J, Haby MM, et al. Cost-effectiveness of cognitive-behavioural therapy and drug interventions for major depression. Aust N Z J Psychiatry 2005;39(8):683-92.

29.   Antonuccio DO, Danton WG, Denelsky GY. Psychotherapy Versus Medication for Depression - Challenging the Conventional Wisdom with Data. Professional Psychology-Research and Practice 1995;26(6):574-585.

30.   Fava GA, Rafanelli C, Grandi S, et al. Six-year outcome for cognitive behavioral treatment of residual symptoms in major depression. Am J Psychiatry 1998;155(10):1443-5.

31.   Hollon SD. Does cognitive therapy have an enduring effect? Cognit Ther Res 2003;27(1):71-75.

32.   Perepletchikova F, Treat TA, Kazdin AE. Treatment integrity in psychotherapy research: analysis of the studies and examination of the associated factors. J Consult Clin Psychol 2007;75(6):829-41.

33.   Beck JS. *Cognitive Therapy: Basics and Beyond.* New York: Guilford Press; 1995.

34.   Weissman MM, Markowitz JC, Klerman GL. *Comprehensive Guide to Interpersonal Psychotherapy* New York: Basic Books; 2000.

35.   Dewan MJ, Steenbarger BN, Greenberg RP, et al. Brief psychotherapies. The American Psychiatric Publishing textbook of psychiatry (5th ed.). Arlington, VA: American Psychiatric Publishing, Inc.; 2008:1154-1170.

36.   Whitlock EP, Lin JS, Chou R, et al. Using existing systematic reviews in complex systematic reviews. Ann Intern Med 2008;148(10):776-82.

37.   Moher D, Cook DJ, Eastwood S, et al. Improving the quality of reports of meta-analyses of randomised controlled trials: the QUOROM statement. Quality of Reporting of Meta-analyses. Lancet 1999;354(9193):1896-900.

38.   Marinopoulos SS, Dorman T, Ratanawongsa N, et al. Effectiveness of Continuing Medical Education. Evidence Report/Technology Assessment No. 149 (Prepared by the Johns Hopkins Evidence-based Practice Center, under Contract No. 290-02-0018.) AHRQ Publication No. 07-E006. Rockville, MD: Agency for Healthcare Research and Quality January 2007. Available at: www.ncbi.nlm.nih.gov/bookshelf/br.fcgi?book=erta149. Accessed January 12, 2011.

39.　　Agency for Healthcare Research and Quality. Methods Guide for Effectiveness and Comparative Effectiveness Reviews. Rockville, MD: Agency for Healthcare Research and Quality. Available at: www.effectivehealthcare.ahrq.gov/index.cfm/search-for-guides-reviews-and-reports/?pageaction=displayproduct&productid=318. Accessed January 12, 2011.

40.　　Cohen J. *Statistical power analysis for the behavioral sciences*. 2nd ed Hillsdale, N.J.: L. Erlbaum Associates; 1988.

41.　　Kraemer HC, Kupfer DJ. Size of treatment effects and their importance to clinical research and practice. Biol Psychiatry 2006;59(11):990-6.

42.　　Borenstein M. *Introduction to meta-analysis* Chichester, West Sussex, U.K. ; Hoboken: John Wiley & Sons; 2009.

43.　　Higgins JP, Thompson SG. Quantifying heterogeneity in a meta-analysis. Stat Med 2002;21(11):1539-58.

44.　　Atkins D, Best D, Briss PA, et al. Grading quality of evidence and strength of recommendations. BMJ 2004;328(7454):1490.

45.　　Cuijpers P, van Straten A, van Schaik A, et al. Psychological treatment of depression in primary care: a meta-analysis. Br J Gen Pract 2009;59(559):e51-60.

46.　　Cape J, Whittington C, Buszewicz M, et al. Brief psychological therapies for anxiety and depression in primary care: meta-analysis and meta-regression. BMC Med 2010;8(1):38.

47.　　Cuijpers P, van Straten A, Warmerdam L, et al. Psychological treatment of depression: a meta-analytic database of randomized studies. BMC Psychiatry 2008;8:36. Available at: (www.psychotherapyrcts.org/index.php?id=3). Accessed January 12, 2011.

48.　　Barrett JE, Williams JW, Jr., Oxman TE, et al. Treatment of dysthymia and minor depression in primary care: a randomized trial in patients aged 18 to 59 years. J Fam Pract 2001;50(5):405-12.

49.　　Lynch DJ, Tamburrino MB, Nagel R. Telephone counseling for patients with minor depression: preliminary findings in a family practice setting. J Fam Pract 1997;44(3):293-8.

50.　　Lynch D, Tamburrino M, Nagel R, et al. Telephone-based treatment for family practice patients with mild depression. Psychol Rep 2004;94(3 Pt 1):785-92.

51.　　Mynors-Wallis LM, Gath DH, Lloyd-Thomas AR, et al. Randomised controlled trial comparing problem solving treatment with amitriptyline and placebo for major depression in primary care. BMJ 1995;310(6977):441-5.

52.　　Scott C, Tacchi MJ, Jones R, et al. Acute and one-year outcome of a randomised controlled trial of brief cognitive therapy for major depressive disorder in primary care. Br J Psychiatry 1997;171:131-4.

53.　　Ward E, King M, Lloyd M, et al. Randomised controlled trial of non-directive counselling, cognitive-behaviour therapy, and usual general practitioner care for patients with depression. I: clinical effectiveness. BMJ 2000;321(7273):1383-8.

54.　　King M, Sibbald B, Ward E, et al. Randomised controlled trial of non-directive counselling, cognitive-behaviour therapy and usual general practitioner care in the management of depression as well as mixed anxiety and depression in primary care. Health Technol Assess 2000;4(19):1-83.

55.　　Williams JW, Jr., Barrett J, Oxman T, et al. Treatment of dysthymia and minor depression in primary care: A randomized controlled trial in older adults. JAMA 2000;284(12):1519-26.

56.　　Barnhofer T, Crane C, Hargus E, et al. Mindfulness-based cognitive therapy as a treatment for chronic depression: A preliminary study. Behav Res Ther 2009;47(5):366-73.

57.　　Laidlaw K, Davidson K, Toner H, et al. A randomised controlled trial of cognitive behaviour therapy vs treatment as usual in the treatment of mild to moderate late life depression. Int J Geriatr Psychiatry 2008;23(8):843-50.

58.　　Mynors-Wallis LM, Gath DH, Day A, et al. Randomised controlled trial of problem solving treatment, antidepressant medication, and combined treatment for major depression in primary care. BMJ 2000;320(7226):26-30.

59.　　Nezu AM. Efficacy of a social problem-solving therapy approach for unipolar depression. J Consult Clin Psychol 1986;54(2):196-202.

60.　　Simon GE, Ludman EJ, Tutty S, et al. Telephone psychotherapy and telephone care management for primary care patients starting antidepressant treatment: a randomized controlled trial. JAMA 2004;292(8):935-42.

61.　　Simon GE, Ludman EJ, Rutter CM. Incremental benefit and cost of telephone care management and telephone psychotherapy for depression in primary care. Arch Gen Psychiatry 2009;66(10):1081-9.

62.　　Wilson PH. Combined pharmacological and behavioural treatment of depression. Behav Res Ther 1982;20(2):173-84.

63.　　Wilson PH. Comparative efficacy of behavioral and cognitive therapies of depression. Cognit Ther Res 1983;7(2):111-124.

64.　　Anonymous. Uniform Mental Health Services in VA Medical Centers and Clinics. VA Handbook 1160.01. Department of Veterans Affairs. Veterans Health Administration. Washington, DC. 2008. Available at: http://www1.va.gov/vhapublications/ViewPublication.asp?pub_ID=1762. Accessed January 12, 2011.

APPENDIX A: SEARCH STRATEGY

Primary Literature (January 2009 through July 2010)

Final limits: Human, Adult, 19+ years, English, Randomized Controlled Trial, Publication date from January 1, 2009 to July 31, 2010.

Step	Terms	Result
1. Replication of Cuijpers database therapy terms	Behavior therapy OR biofeedback OR cognitive analytic therapy PR counseling OR family therapy PR marital therapy PR psychoanalytic therapy OR psychotherapy PR relaxation therapy	1822
2. Replication of Cuijpers database depression terms	"depressive disorder"[MeSH Terms] OR ("depressive"[All Fields] AND "disorder"[All Fields]) OR "depressive disorder"[All Fields] OR "depression"[All Fields] OR "depression"[MeSH Terms] OR depressive[All Fields]	1152
3. Addition of other terms for types of therapy of interest for this report	Interpersonal therapy OR problem-solving therapy OR mindfulness-based cognitive therapy OR cognitive behavioral analysis system of psychotherapy OR dialectical behavior therapy OR functional analytic psychotherapy OR acceptance and commitment therapy	178
4. Final search	(#1 OR #3) AND #2	383

Systematic Reviews

Final limits: English, All Adult: 19+ years, Systematic Reviews, Publication date from 2000.

Step	Terms	Result
1	Search (("depressive symptoms"[All Fields]) OR ("Depression"[Mesh] OR "Depressive Disorder"[Mesh]) OR (depression))	51523
2	Search (minor AND depression) OR (subthreshold AND depression) OR (subsyndromal AND depression)	3689
3	Search major depressive disorder[mesh]	64244
4	Search dysthymia OR dysthymic disorder[mesh]	2407
5	Search adjustment disorder[mesh]	3615
6	Search 1 OR 2 OR 3 OR 4 OR 5	69903
7	Search ((cognitive behavioral therapy OR CBT OR cognitive therapy OR behavior therapy OR interpersonal therapy OR IPT OR problem-solving therapy OR PST OR mindfulness-based cognitive therapy OR MBCT OR ("cognitive behavioral analysis system" AND therapy) OR CBASP OR dialectical behavioral therapy OR DBT OR functional analytic psychotherapy OR FAP OR (acceptance AND commitment AND therapy) OR ACT OR short-term psychodynamic therapy) OR (psychotherapy, brief[mesh]))	297485
8	Search Cochrane Database Syst Rev [TA] OR search[Title/Abstract] OR meta-analysis[Publication Type] OR MEDLINE[Title/abstract] OR (systematic[Title/Abstract] AND review[Title/Abstract])	159125
9	Search 6 AND 7 AND 8	341

APPENDIX B: EVIDENCE TABLES

BRIEF PSYCHOTHERAPY FOR DEPRESSION IN PRIMARY CARE

Study ID: Barnhofer, Crane, Hargus, et al., 2009

Study Information	Participants	Interventions	Results and Adverse Effects	Comments/ Quality Scoring
Geographical location: Oxford, England	**Age:** Mean (SD): 42 MBCT: 42.07 (11.34) TAU: 41.79 (9.52) Median: NR Range: 18 to 65	**Intervention description:** RCT of 2 arms: 1. MBCT: 14 participants 2. TAU: 14 participants	**Eligible randomized:** 31 of 34 (91%)	**General comments:** Stats were LOCF – now frowned upon in favor of modeling or imputation
Recruitment method: - Advertisement - Referral	**Education:** Mean (SD) MBCT: 16.38 (3.04) TAU: 15.21 (3.19)	**Depression intervention(s):** Behavioral intervention Type: MBCT for 8 sessions of 2-hr duration delivered via manual (Segal, 2002) modified for suicidality with homework of mindfulness practice 1 hr per day, 6 days per wk	**Followup rate:** Total: 28 of 31 (90%) MCBT: 14 of 16 (86%) TAU: 15 of 16 (94%)	**Study-level quality assessment:** Good
Recruitment setting: - Mental health - Nonclinical	**Sex:** Female n (%): 19 of 28 (68%) MBCT: 10 of 14 (71%) TAU: 9 of 14 (64%)	Delivery: Group Intensity: 8 weekly 2 hr Fidelity monitoring: Yes	**Important baseline differences:** Presence of chronic depression higher in TAU (n = 12) versus MBCT (n = 7), p = 0.04	**Assessment of adverse effects adequate?** Yes
Treatment setting: - Mental health - Academic	**Race/ethnicity:** NR	Other notes about intervention: All on some type of antidepressant	**Depression outcomes:** BDI-II	**Applicability:** - High education - Mostly women
Study design: RCT	**Veterans:** NR	**Therapist** Discipline: CBT Experience: NR Training: internship at the Center for Mindfulness in Medicine, University of Massachusetts	Response rates n (%): BDI fell to < 13 MBCT: 6 (37) TAU: 1 (6) P = 0.04	
Number of participants enrolled: 31	**Baseline depression assessment(s):** Criterion: DSM-IV Disorder: Chronic MDD n (%) MBCT: 7 (50%) TAU: 12 (85%)	**Comparator:** Behavioral control Type: TAU Delivery: Mixed Intensity: Mixed Fidelity monitoring: No	Change in diagnosis: MBCT: 7 of 10 TAU: 2 of 11 P = 0.03	
Duration of followup: 8 wk	Current: 100% Severity score: mean (SD) MBCT: 29.36 (9.66) TAU: 31.32 (10.79) Chronicity: 20+ years for current	Other notes about control: All on some type of antidepressant	Severity score: mean (SD) MBCT: 17.62 (10.94) TAU: 28.86 (12.97)	
	Prior episodes: At least 3 prior episodes lasting 2 yr	**Cointervention—psychotropic drugs:** None	**HRQOL outcomes:** NR **Other outcomes:** Social: No Occupational: No Satisfaction: No Suicidal ideation: Yes	

Study ID: Barnhofer, Crane, Hargus, et al., 2009

Study Information	Participants	Interventions	Results and Adverse Effects	Comments/ Quality Scoring

	Comorbid psychiatric conditions: N (%)
	 Alcohol/substance abuse: Excluded
	 Anxiety disorder:
	   MBCT: 4 (28%)
	   TAU: 6 (42%)
	 PTSD: NR
	 Other:
	   Suicide attempt: 8 (56%)
	   MBCT: 4 (28%)
	   TAU: 4 (28%)
	
	 Comorbid chronic medical conditions: NR
	
	 Inclusion criteria:
	 1. History of 3 episodes MDD
	 2. Current MDD or subthreshold MDD
	 3. History of suicidality
	 4. Absence of other severe mental health diagnosis, especially self-harm
	 5. Adequate written and oral English
	 6. Not currently in treatment
	 7. Ages 18 to 65
	
	 Exclusion criteria: NR
			Treatment discontinuation rate: 3 (9.7%)
			
			 Adverse effects: None reported related to intervention	

Brief Psychotherapy for Depression in Primary Care

Study ID: Laidlaw, Davidson, Toner, et al., 2008

Study Information	Participants	Interventions	Results and Adverse Effects	Comments/Quality Scoring

Study Information

Geographical location: UK (Fife and Glasgow)

Recruitment method: Referral

Recruitment setting: Primary care

Treatment setting:
- Unclear
- Nonacademic

Study design: RCT

Number of participants enrolled: 44

Duration of followup: 6 mo

Participants

Age:
Mean (SD)
CBT: 74 (8.39)
TAU: 74.05 (7.62)
Median: NR
Range: NR

Education:
Mean (SD)
CBT: 10.10 (1.74)
TAU: 9.9 (1.29)

Sex:
Female n (%):
CBT: 11 (60%)
TAU: 18 (85%)

Race/ethnicity: NR

Veterans: NR

Baseline depression assessment(s):
BDI ns
CBT: 19.6 (5.22)
TAU: 19.5 (5.48)
GDS ns
CBT: 7.6 (2.7)
TAU: 8.5 (3.55)
HAM-D ns
CBT: 11.4 (3.08)
TAU: 11.8 (2.84)
Disorder: MDD
Severity: NR
Chronicity: NR
Prior episodes: NR

Interventions

Intervention description:
Two arms:
1. CBT: 21 participants
2. TAU: 23 participants

CBT followed conceptual model and protocol developed by Beck. TAU was as close to standard care as possible. No restrictions on type of treatment; also, no treatment was allowed if GP thought appropriate.

Depression intervention(s):
Behavioral intervention
Type: CBT
Delivery: Mean 8 sessions (SD = 4.7, range 2 to 17)
Intensity: NR (assumed weekly since adhering to Beck's protocol)
Fidelity monitoring: Yes, audiotaped and rated with Cognitive Therapy Rating Scale by cognitive therapy experts

Other notes about intervention: Assumption is that the sessions were weekly given that they said they adhered to Beck's model, in which case post results should approximate 8 sessions; however, frequency of sessions not provided.

Therapist
Discipline: Psychology
Experience: NR
Training: Master's level (except for one who was graduate level with several years of experience)

Results and Adverse Effects

Eligible randomized: 61% (based on Figure 1, 115 referred, 28 + 44 eligible, 44 randomized)

Followup rate: 40 (90.9%)

Important baseline differences: Gender (TAU had higher percentage of female; CBT had higher percentage of male)

Depression outcomes:
Response rates:
CBT: 20
TAU: 20

BDI

	CBT	TAU	F, p
Post treatment	9.4 (8.56)	13.25 (10.3)	1.65 0.21
3 mo	9 (8.16)	12.9 (9.34)	1.98 0.17
6 mo	10.55 (9.05)	15.10 (11.83)	1.87 0.18

GDS

	CBT	TAU	F, p
Post treatment	3.85 (3.83)	5.3 (3.48)	1.57 0.22
3 mo	5 (3.71)	4.9 (3.35)	0.008 0.93
6 mo	5.05 (3.46)	5.75 (3.72)	0.38 0.54

Comments/Quality Scoring

General comments:
- Adequate randomization
- Missing data adequately addressed
- Blinding not possible given intervention but assessors were blinded
- No concerns regarding selective outcome reporting
- No conflicts of interest

Study-level quality assessment
Fair

Comments:
- Small sample size
- Missing information from the protocol that would allow evaluation of applicability to our question

Assessment of adverse effects adequate?
Unclear

Applicability:
To general population:
Yes

To Veterans: Yes

Limitations:
- Not enough information on disease severity
- Intensity of therapy not given
- UK primary care may differ from US

Study ID: Laidlaw, Davidson, Toner, et al., 2008

Study Information	Participants	Interventions	Results and Adverse Effects	Comments/ Quality Scoring

Participants

Comorbid psychiatric conditions:
N (%)
Alcohol/substance abuse: NR
PTSD: NR
Other anxiety disorder: NR
Other: Axis I disorder: CBT-2 (10%), 6 (30%)

Comorbid chronic medical conditions:
Mean (SD)
  CBT: 2.26 (1.2)
  TAU: 2.2 (0.83)
Conditions not specified

Inclusion criteria:
1. Age 60 or over
2. Met DSM-IV criteria for MDD using the SADS-L structured interview
3. HAM-D = 7-24
4. BDI-II = 13 to 28
5. Can provide written consent
6. Not prescribed antidepression medication within 3 mo of referral to trial

Exclusion criteria:
1. Insufficient knowledge of English
2. MMSE < 22
3. Received more than 6 sessions of CBT in the past or currently receiving psychological therapy

Interventions

Comparator:
Behavioral control
Type: TAU
Delivery: Standard care
Intensity: At GP's discretion
Fidelity monitoring: Yes, checking GP notes at the end of study and asking participants about treatment received; however, no adherence data since there were guidelines given to GPs

Other notes about control: 16 (80%) received medications

Cointervention—psychotropic drugs:
Drug name/dose: None provided by the study
Clinician discipline: NA

Results and Adverse Effects

HAM-D

	CBT	TAU	F, p
Post treatment	5.25 (4.48)	7.75 (6.05)	2.2 0.15
3 mo	5.15 (4.75)	6.7 (6.23)	.78 0.38
6 mo	6.7 (5.03)	7.55 (6.13)	.23 0.63

HRQOL outcomes:
WHOQOL Physical Subscale

	CBT	TAU	F, p
Post treatment	22.4 (5.02)	19.85 (4.34)	0.29 0.59
3 mo	21.6 (3.66)	20.75 (5.3)	0.02 0.9
6 mo	21.35 (5.34)	20 (5.69)	.0.75 0.39

WHOQOL Psychological Subscale

	CBT	TAU	F, p
Post treatment	20.65 (3.13)	18.15 (3.66)	0.14 0.71
3 mo	19.65 (2.62)	19.15 (3.13)	0.08 0.78
6 mo	19.2 (3.43)	17.75 (3.99)	2.39 0.13

Other outcomes:
Social: WHOQOL Social Relationships

	CBT	TAU	F, p
Post treatment	10.05 (2.66)	9.95 (1.4)	1.72 0.09
3 mo	11 (1.26)	10.55 (1.23)	0.35 0.56
6 mo	10.5 (1.4)	10.2 (1.47)	0.77 0.44

Study ID: Laidlaw, Davidson, Toner, et al., 2008

Study Information	Participants	Interventions	Results and Adverse Effects	Comments/ Quality Scoring
			Occupational: NR Satisfaction: NR **Treatment discontinuation rate**: Withdrew from study at 6 mo followup: CBT: 2 TAU: 4 **Adverse effects**: NR	

Brief Psychotherapy for Depression in Primary Care

Study ID: Mynors-Wallis, Gath, Day, et al., 2000

Study Information	Participants	Interventions	Results and Adverse Effects	Comments/ Quality Scoring
Geographical location: Oxfordshire, UK	**Age:** Mean (SD) Med: 34 (NR) MedPST: 35 (NR) Median: NR Med range: 19 to 58 MedPST range: 19 to 62	**Intervention description:** Four arms: 1. Problem-solving treatment (PST) alone provided by GP (excluded from this analysis): 39 participants 2. PST alone provided by nurse (excluded from this analysis): 41 participants 3. Medication alone (Med): 36 participants 4. Medication + PST (MedPST) provided by nurse: 35 participants	**Eligible randomized:** 83% **Followup rate:** N (%) Med 6 wk: 34 of 36 (94%) MedPST 6 wk: 34 of 35 (97%) Med 12 wk: 34 of 36 (94%) MedPST 12 wk: 31 of 35 (89%) Med 52 wk: 30 of 36 (83%) MedPST 52 wk: 30 of 35 (86%)	**General comments:** PST alone (provided by either GP or nurse) found to be equally efficacious to medication alone, and addition of PST to medication did not result in significant benefit
Recruitment method: Referral	**Education:** N (%) Med: 9 (25%) > 16 yr MedPST: 8 (23%) > 16 yr			**Study-level quality assessment** Good
Recruitment setting: Primary care	**Sex:** Female n (%) Med: 31 (86%) MedPST: 24 (69%)	**Depression intervention(s):** Behavioral intervention Type: MedPST; PST for use in primary care settings was added to GP prescription of fluvoxamine or paroxetine Delivery: Individual Intensity: 6 sessions (first session, 1 hr; rest 30 min) over 12 wk Fidelity monitoring: No	**Important baseline differences:** None **Depression outcomes:** HRSD Recovered (HRSD ≤ 7): Med 12 wk: 24 (67%) MedPST 12 wk: 21 (60%)	**Assessment of adverse effects adequate?** Yes; research interviewers were blind
Treatment setting: - Primary care (i.e., patients' home or local health center) - Nonacademic	**Race/ethnicity:** White n (%) Med: 32 (89%) MedPST: 34 (97%)		Med 52 wk: 20 (56%) MedPST 52 wk: 23 (66%)	**Applicability:** To general population: - Comorbid conditions not reported - Therapists likely more skilled than typical providers - UK treatment settings different than typical US primary care
Study design: RCT	**Veterans:** No	**Therapist** Discipline: Research practice nurse Experience: Participated in previous study as problem-solving therapist Training: Nursing; trained in PST by study investigator	Severity score mean (95% CI): Med 12 wk: 6.2 (3.7 to 8.6) MedPST 12 wk: 7.5 (5.2 to 9.9) Med 52 wk: 7.2 (5.1 to 9.2) MedPST 52 wk: 5.7 (3.4 to 7.9)	
Number of participants enrolled: 71	**Baseline depression assessment(s):** Criterion: HRSD ≥ 13 Disorder: 71 (100%) probable or definite MDD	**Comparator:** Behavioral control Type: Med; GP prescribed fluvoxamine or paroxetine in accordance with practice guidelines Delivery: Individual Intensity: NR Fidelity monitoring: No	BDI mean (95% CI) Med 12 wk: 11.8 (7.8 to 15.8) MedPST 12 wk: 9.3 (6.6 to 12.0) Med 52 wk: 11.5 (6.9 to 16.2) MedPST 52 wk: 8.6 (5.3 to 11.9)	**To Veterans:** - Patient sample predominantly female - From UK - Treatment often provided in home
Duration of followup: 52 wk	HRSD mean (95% CI) Med: 20.2 (19.1 to 21.4) MedPST: 19.8 (18.5 to 21.1) BDI mean (95% CI) Med: 30.2 (27.7 to 32.7) MedPST: 30.0 (27.3 to 32.6)		CIS mean (95% CI) Med 12 wk: 9.8 (6.1 to 13.5) MedPST 12 wk: 9.6 (6.3 to 12.9) Med 52 wk: 11.5 (7.3 to 5.6) MedPST 52 wk: 9.7 (5.9 to 13.6)	

Study ID: Mynors-Wallis, Gath, Day, et al., 2000

Study Information	Participants	Interventions	Results and Adverse Effects	Comments/ Quality Scoring
	CIS-D mean (95% CI) Med: 29.3 (27.3 to 31.2) MedPST: 29.0 (26.5 to 31.5) Chronicity: Med 12 (33%) > 6 mo MedPST: 13 (37%) > 6mo Prior episodes: Med ≥ 1: 19(53%) MedPST ≥ 1: 19(54%) **Comorbid psychiatric conditions:** Alcohol/substance abuse: NR (excluded) PTSD: NR (excludec) Other anxiety disorder: NR (excluded) **Comorbid chronic medical conditions:** NR **Inclusion criteria:** 1. GP suspected MDD 2. Probable or definite MDD on research diagnostic criteria 3. HRSD ≥ 13 4. MDD duration ≥ 4 wk **Exclusion criteria:** 1. Psychiatric disorcer preceding MDD cnset 2. Concurrent MDD treatment 3. Brain damage 4. Learning difficulties 5. Schizophrenia 6. Drug dependence 7. Recent alcohol abuse 8. Physical illness 9. MDD with psychotic features or suicidal intent	**Cointervention—psychotropic drugs :** Drug name/dose : Fluvoxamine/initial dose 100 mg ; or paroxetine/initial dose 20 mg Clinician discipline : GP	**HRQOL outcomes:** None **Other outcomes:** Social: Yes (social adjustment scale) Occupational: No Satisfaction: No **Treatment discontinuation rate:** Med: 6 (17%) MedPST: 6 (17%) **Adverse effects:** N (%) Med medication side effects: 2 (6%) MedPST medication side effects: 4 (11%)	

Brief Psychotherapy for Depression in Primary Care

Study ID: Nezu, 1986

Study Information	Participants	Interventions	Results and Adverse Effects	Comments/Quality Scoring
Geographical location: USA **Recruitment method:** Advertisement **Recruitment setting:** Nonclinical (ad) **Treatment setting:** - **Mental health** - Academic (university psychology clinic) **Study design:** RCT **Number of participants enrolled: 21** **Duration of followup:** - 8 wk for PST vs WLC - 6 mo for PST vs PFT	**Age:** Mean (SD): 41.73 (12.81) Median: NR Range: NR **Education:** Mean (SD): 15.96 (2.59) yr **Sex:** Female n (%): PST: 10 (83%) WLC: 7 (78%) **Race/ethnicity: NR** **Veterans: No** **Baseline depression assessment(s):** Criterion: Research Diagnostic Criteria Disorder: 21 (100%) MDD BDI PST: 23.91 (7.09) WLC: 20.67 (5.39) MMPI-D PST: 81.36 (8.12) WLC: 78.76 (7.05) Chronicity: NR Prior episodes: NR **Comorbid psychiatric conditions:** Alcohol/substance abuse: NR (exclusion criterion) PTSD: NR Other anxiety disorder: NR Other: NR	**Intervention description:** Three arms: 1. Problem-focused therapy (PFT) (excluded from this analysis): 11 participants 2. Problem-solving therapy (PST): 12 participants 3. Waitlist control (WLC): 9 participants **Depression intervention(s):** <u>Behavioral intervention</u> Type: PST based on D'Zurrila and Nezu's (1982) five-component model Delivery: Group Intensity: 8 weekly 1.5 to 2 hr sessions Fidelity monitoring: Partial (weekly supervision to ensure adherence to relevant treatment manuals) Other notes about behavioral intervention: Therapist allegiance very likely a confound for PST vs PFT but not for PST vs waitlist <u>Therapist</u> Discipline: Two psychology graduate students Experience: Average 4.5 years supervised psychotherapy experience Training: Prior training in group therapy and PST model; weekly supervision from author during treatment period	**Eligible randomized:** 78% **Followup rate:** N (%) PST 8 wk: 11 of 12 (92%) WLC 8 wk: 6 of 9 (67%) (3 excluded because entered therapy in interim) PST 6 mo: 10 of 12 (83%) **Important baseline differences:** None **Depression outcomes:** BDI PST 8 wk: 9.82 (4.71) WLC 8 wk: 21.00 (6.27) PST 6 mo: 9.50 (3.64) MMPI-D PST 8 wk: 54.27 (4.62) WLC 8 wk: 76.33 (4.89) PST 6 mo: 52.50 (6.89) **HRQOL outcomes:** None **Other outcomes:** Social: No Occupational: No Satisfaction: No **Treatment discontinuation rate:** PST: 1 (8%) **Adverse effects:** NR	**General comments:** Therapist allegiance to and experience in PST both very high **Study-level quality assessment** Fair Comments: - 33% of WLC excluded from analysis because sought treatment - Outcome assessors were not blind (although clinical interview not used as outcome measure) - Therapist allegiance to PST likely very high **Assessment of adverse effects adequate?** No **Applicability:** <u>To general population:</u> - Patients recruited through newspaper ads - Therapist skill in and adherence to PST higher than typical clinician - Intensive treatment for PC setting

Study ID: Nezu, 1986

Study Information	Participants	Interventions	Results and Adverse Effects	Comments/ Quality Scoring
	Comorbid chronic medical conditions: NR **Inclusion criteria:** 1. Responded to advertisement 2. BDI ≥ 16 3. Depressive episode ≥ 4 weeks 4. Meet Research Diagnostic Criteria for MDD 5. MMPI-D T score > 70 **Exclusion criteria:** 1. Mental retardation 2. Psychotic symptomatology 3. Active substance use 4. Organic brain syndrome 5. Current MDD treatment	**Comparator:** Behavioral control Type: WLC invited to receive treatment at the end of 8-wk program Delivery: NA Intensity: NA Fidelity monitoring: No **Cointervention—psychotropic drugs:** None		To Veterans: - Patient sample predominantly female - Comorbid conditions not reported - University psychology clinic setting

41

Brief Psychotherapy for Depression in Primary Care

Study ID: Simon, Ludman, Tutty, et al., 2004, and Simon, Ludman, and Rutter, 2009

Study Information	Participants	Interventions	Results and Adverse Effects	Comments/Quality Scoring
Geographical location: Washington State and Northern Idaho, USA	**Age:** Mean (SD) Usual care: 44.0 (16.0) Care management (CM): 44.9 (15.3) Psychotherapy + CM: 44.7 (15.7) Median: NR Range: NR	**Intervention description:** Three arms: 1. Telephone-based psychotherapy (CBT) + CM: 195 participants 2. Telephone CM: 207 participants 3. Usual care: 195 participants	**Eligible randomized:** 95% **Followup rate:** N (%): 578 (96%) had 1 followup 532 (89%) completed 6 month followup	**General comments:** None **Study-level quality assessment:** Good
Recruitment method: Registry (Group Health Cooperative membership)	**Education:** College graduate: 39.3%	**Depression intervention(s):** Behavioral intervention Type: CBT; 8 sessions structured assessment, motivational enhancement, behavioral activation, cognitive restructuring, self-care plan Delivery: Telephone Intensity: 8 sessions 30 to 40 min; first four sessions every wk, second four 1 to 4 wk apart Fidelity monitoring: No	CM: 97% had 1 contact 85% had 3 contacts Psychotherapy + CM: 14 (7%) had no sessions 2 (1%) had 1 session only 167 (84%) had ≥ 4 sessions 125 (25%) had ≥ 7 sessions	**Comments:** - Comparable groups - Little missing data - Outcome assessors blinded - Not free of selective outcome reporting - PHQ results not reported - SCL scores at outcome not reported
Recruitment setting: Primary care	**Sex:** Female: 74.33%		**Important baseline differences:** None	**Assessment of adverse effects adequate?** NR
Treatment setting: Primary care	**Race/ethnicity:** White: 80% **Veterans:** NR	**Other notes about intervention:** Psychotherapy was in addition to CM	**Depression outcomes:** 6-mo followup using SCL (50% reduction)	**Applicability:** -Severity of baseline depression, chronicity and comorbid condition not given
Study design: RCT	**Baseline depression assessment:** Criterion: Hopkins Symptom Checklist (SCL) Disorder: NR Severity: mean (SD) Usual Care: 1.55 (0.62) CM: 1.54 (0.61) Psychotherapy + CM: 1.52 (0.59) Chronicity: NR Prior episodes: NR	**Therapist** Discipline: Master's-level psychologist Experience: At least 1 yr clinical experience Training: 12 hr didactic and role play, observation, and audiotaping of 6 sessions each, 1 hr weekly supervision, twice monthly motivational interviewing seminar	Response rates n (%): Usual care: 76 of 176 (43%) CM: 94 of 184 (51%) Psychotherapy + CM: 100 of 172 (58%) Severity score: NR	- Sample was from a group model primary care clinic who did not want referral to mental health clinic - CM involved significant outreach (at least 5 phone calls) per participant, which is not routine clinical practice
Number of participants enrolled: 600				
Duration of followup: 6 wk, 12 wk, and 24 wk	**Comorbid psychiatric conditions:** NR Alcohol/substance abuse: NR Anxiety disorder: NR PTSD: NR Other: NR			

Brief Psychotherapy for Depression in Primary Care

Study ID: Simon, Ludman, Tutty, et al., 2004, and Simon, Ludman, and Rutter, 2009

Study Information	Participants	Interventions	Results and Adverse Effects	Comments/ Quality Scoring
	Comorbid chronic medical conditions: NR **Inclusion criteria:** 1. Beginning antidepressant 2. SCL Score > 0.5 **Exclusion criteria:** 1. Not a new episode of antidepressant treatment 2. Bipolar 3. Schizophrenia 4. Planning or receiving psychotherapy 5. Cognitive, language, or hearing impairment	**Comparator 1:** **Behavioral control** Type: Usual care; any treatment normally available including primary care physician visits and referral to mental health Delivery: NR Intensity: NR Fidelity monitoring: No **Comparator 2:** Behavioral control Type: Telephone CM; assessment of depression, antidepressant use, and adverse effects. Scripts for addressing concerns and motivational enhancement. Primary care physicians received summary and computer-generated recommendations. Also care coordination, outreach, and as-needed crisis intervention. Delivery: Telephone Intensity: Wk 4, 12, 20 Fidelity monitoring: No **Cointervention—psychotropic drugs:** NR	**HRQOL outcomes:** NR **Other outcomes:** NNT 6.4 for 50% reduction in SCL psychotherapy + CM versus usual care Social: NR Occupational: NR Satisfaction: Self-rated "very satisfied"— Usual care: 50 of 176 (29%) CM: 85 of 184 (47%) Psychotherapy + CM: 101 of 172 (59%) Self-rated "much improved"— Usual care: 97 of 176 (55%) CM: 121 of 184 (66%) Psychotherapy + CM: 100 of 172 (58%) Total depression costs: $ Mean (SD) Usual care: 1020 (1009) CM: 1485 (1258) Psychotherapy + CM:1670 (1110) Total health care costs $ Mean (SD) Usual care: 9406 (10554) CM: 10268 (9773) Psychotherapy + CM: 9334 (8432) **Treatment discontinuation rate:** N (%) 14 (7%) had no sessions 2 (1%) had 1 session only 167 (84%) had ≥ 4 sessions 125 (25%) had ≥ 7 sessions **Adverse effects:** NR	

Brief Psychotherapy for Depression in Primary Care

Study ID: Wilson, 1982

Study Information	Participants	Interventions	Results and Adverse Effects	Comments/ Quality Scoring
Geographical location: Sydney, Australia	**Age:** Mean (SD): 38.8 (NR) Median: NR Range: 20 to 55	**Intervention description:** Patients randomly allocated within sex to: 1. Amitriptyline +task assignment 2. Amitriptyline + relaxation therapy 3. Amitriptyline+ minimal contact 4. Placebo +task assignment 5. Placebo+ relaxation therapy 6. Placebo + minimal contact	**Eligible randomized:** 97; 64 analyzed in completers analysis	**General comments:** None
Recruitment method: Advertisement	**Education:** NR		**Followup rate:** 64 (65.9%)	**Study-level quality assessment** Poor
Recruitment setting: Mental health	**Sex:** Female: 42 (65.6%) **Race/ethnicity:** NR		**Important baseline differences:** None	**Comments:** - Unclear randomization - Unclear allocation concealment
Treatment setting: Academic	**Veterans:** None **Baseline depression assessment(s):** Criterion: BDI Disorder: NR	**Depression intervention(s):** Behavioral intervention Type: Behavioral therapy, 7 sessions over 1 hr Delivery: Individual Intensity: NR Fidelity monitoring: NR	**Depression outcomes:** 8 wk: Placebo +task assignment: 11.89 (10.87) Placebo+ relaxation therapy: 16.55 (10.36) Placebo + minimal contact: 14.67 (11.12)	- Incomplete data not addressed - Unclear blinding (not blinded to drug) - Selective outcome reporting
Study design: RCT, stratified by sex	Severity: Amitriptyline +task assignment: 26.08 (7.61) Amitriptyline + relaxation therapy: 23.10 (3.51)		6 mo: Placebo +task assignment: 10.00 (8.14) Placebo+ relaxation therapy: 11.27 (7.98) Placebo + minimal contact: 15.18 (10.86)	**Assessment of adverse effects adequate?** No
Number of participants enrolled: 97, 64 analyzed	Amitriptyline+ minimal contact: 25.8 (5.12) Placebo +task assignment: 27.22 (4.87)	**Other notes about intervention:** Adapted from MacPhillamy and Lewinsohn therapy		**Applicability:** To general population: - Done in Australia - University setting - Recruitment via advertising
Duration of followup: - 8 wk - 6 mo posttrial followup	Placebo+ relaxation therapy: 25.82 (4.47) Placebo + minimal contact: 25.00 (5.77)	**Therapist** Discipline: Psychology Experience: Graduate students Training: Previous experience with behavioral treatments (experimental and clinical) not specified further	**Response rates:** NR **Severity score:** NR **HRQOL outcomes:** NR	
	Chronicity: NR Prior episodes: "Past psychological issues in 86%"	**Comparator:** Behavioral control Type: Minimal contact, participants described their problems, nondirective and no specific suggestions Delivery: Individual Intensity: Two 1-hr sessions Fidelity monitoring: NR	**Other outcomes:** Social: No Occupational: No Satisfaction: No	**To Veterans:** - 65% women - Comorbidities NR - Chronicity NR
	Comorbid psychiatric conditions: NR **Comorbid chronic medical conditions:** NR		**Treatment discontinuation rate:** NR **Adverse effects:** NR	

Study ID: Wilson, 1982

Study Information	Participants	Interventions	Results and Adverse Effects	Comments/ Quality Scoring
	Inclusion criteria: 1. BDI ≥ 20 2. Depression ≥ 2 months (self-report) **Exclusion criteria:** 1. No other major psychiatric disorders 2. Not getting any psychological or pharmacological treatments (apart from minor tranquilizers) 3. No contraindications to amitriptyline	Other notes about control: Described as a way for subjects to talk about their problems and see a solution to it themselves **Cointervention—psychotropic drugs:** Drug name/dose: Randomized to drug or placebo. Amitriptyline 50 mg titrated to 150 mg over 6 wk and then titrated off over 6 days Clinician discipline: NR		

Brief Psychotherapy for Depression in Primary Care

Study ID: Wilson, 1983

Study Information	Participants	Interventions	Results and Adverse Effects	Comments/ Quality Scoring
Geographical location: Sydney, Australia	**Age:** Mean : 39.5 Median: NR Range: 20 to 58	**Intervention description:** 1. Behavioral therapy: 8 participants 2. Cognitive therapy: 8 participants 3. Waitlist: 9 participants	**Eligible randomized:** 29	**General comments:** None
Recruitment method: Advertisement	**Education:** 19 (76%) completed at least lower secondary school	**Depression intervention 1:** Behavioral intervention Type: Behavioral activation based on Lewinsohn et al. To increase the frequency, quality, and range of activities and social interactions; mood record also maintained. Delivery: Individual Intensity: Eight 1-hr weekly sessions Fidelity monitoring: No	**Followup rate:** NA; 3 participants in behavioral treatment and 1 in cognitive treatment dropped out and were replaced by new participants	**Study-level quality assessment** Fair **Comments:** - Unclear randomization - Unclear allocation concealment - Unclear blinding - No selective outcome reporting
Recruitment setting: - Mental health, primary care, mixed - Nonclinical	**Sex:** Female: 20 (80%) **Race/ethnicity:** NR		**Important baseline differences:** NR **Depression outcomes:** Response rates: NR Severity scores: BDI	- Patients who dropped out were replaced; possibly not randomized - Comorbidities NR - Limited information reported, but an old study
Treatment setting: - Mental health outpatient - Academic	**Veterans:** No **Baseline depression assessment(s):** - 7 participants had past hospitalization - 2 on antidepressants - 3 on minor tranquilizers	**Depression intervention 2:** Cognitive intervention Type: Cognitive restructuring based on Beck et al. Negative cognitive distortions and irrational beliefs evaluated and positive thought schedule developed for 3 times a day use; thought record also maintained. Delivery: Individual Intensity: Eight 1-hr weekly sessions Fidelity monitoring: No	Behavioral therapy Pre Rx: 21.13 (7.62) Post Rx: 7.50 (4.55) Cognitive therapy Pre Rx: 27.25 (3.80) Post Rx : 9.00 (6.82) Waitlist Pre Rx : 23.66 (7.45) Post Rx: 21.44 (5.52)	**Assessment of adverse effects adequate?** No **Applicability:** To general population: - Recruited via advertising - Treated in Australia - Treatment in a university setting
Study design: RCT **Number of participants enrolled:** 25	Behavioral therapy arm Criterion: BDI Disorder: NR Severity: 21.13 (7.62) Chronicity: At least 3 mo Prior episodes: NR Criterion: HAM-D (17 item)	**Therapist** Discipline: NR Experience: NR Training: NR	HAM-D Behavioral therapy Pre Rx: 13.89 (3.22) Post Rx: 5.25 (3.46)	To Veterans: - 80% women - No comorbidities reported including substance abuse - Dropouts replaced
Duration of followup: - 8 wk - Naturalistic followup of interventions at 30 wk	Disorder: NR Severity: 13.89 (3.22) Chronicity: at least 3 mo Prior episodes: NR	**Comparator:** Behavioral control Type: Waitlist only; no interaction Delivery: None Intensity: None Fidelity monitoring: No **Cointervention—psychotropic drugs:** NR	Cognitive therapy Pre Rx: 13.62 (2.40) Post Rx: 5.88 (5.01) Waitlist Pre Rx: 13.22 (4.08) Post Rx: 14.78 (5.96) **HRQOL outcomes:** NR **Other outcomes:** Social: No Occupational: No Satisfaction: No	

Study ID: Wilson, 1983

Study Information	Participants	Interventions	Results and Adverse Effects	Comments/ Quality Scoring
	Cognitive therapy arm Criterion: BDI Disorder: NR Severity: 27.25 (3.30) Chronicity: At least 3 mo Prior episodes: NR Criterion: HAM-D (17 item) Disorder: NR Severity: 13.62 (2.40) Chronicity: At least 3 mo Prior episodes: NR	Waitlist Criterion: BDI Disorder: NR Severity: 23.66 (7.45) Chronicity: at least 3 mo Prior episodes: NR Criterion: HAM-D (17 item) Disorder: NR Severity: 13.62 (4.08) Chronicity: At least 3 mo Prior episodes: NR **Comorbid psychiatric conditions:** Excluded Alcohol/substance abuse: NR PTSD: NR Other anxiety disorder: NR Other: NR **Comorbid chronic medical conditions:** NR **Inclusion criteria:** 1. BDI ≥ 17 2. Frequent episodes of depression (self-report) 3. Depression for at least 3 mo (self-report) **Exclusion criteria:** 1. Previous/concurrent use of major tranquilizers or lithium 2. No other major physical or psychiatric disorders 3. No suicidal ideation	**Treatment discontinuation rate:** 3 of 8 (37.5%) participants in behavioral treatment and 1 of 8 (12%) in cognitive treatment dropped out and were replaced by new participants **Adverse effects:** NR	

Abbreviations: AE = adverse effects, BDI-II = Beck Depression Inventory-II, CBT = cognitive behavioral therapy, CES-D = Center for Epidemiologic Studies-Depression Scale, CI = confidence interval, DIS = Diagnostic Interview Schedule, HDRS = Hamilton Depression Rating Scale, MDD = major depressive disorder, n = number, NA = not applicable, NR = not reported, ns = not significant, OR = odds ratio, p = probability, PHQ = Patient Health Questionnaire, RCT = randomized controlled trial, SD = standard deviation, SE = standard error, ST = standard treatment, vs = versus, wk = week/weeks, yr = year/years

LIST OF INCLUDED STUDIES FROM PRIMARY LITERATURE IN ALPHABETICAL ORDER

Barnhofer T, Crane C, Hargus E, et al. Mindfulness-based cognitive therapy as a treatment for chronic depression: A preliminary study. Behav Res Ther 2009;47(5):366-73.

Laidlaw K, Davidson K, Toner H, et al. A randomised controlled trial of cognitive behaviour therapy vs treatment as usual in the treatment of mild to moderate late life depression. Int J Geriatr Psychiatry 2008;23(8):843-50.

Mynors-Wallis LM, Gath DH, Day A, et al. Randomised controlled trial of problem solving treatment, antidepressant medication, and combined treatment for major depression in primary care. BMJ 2000;320(7226):26-30.

Nezu AM. Efficacy of a social problem-solving therapy approach for unipolar depression. J Consult Clin Psychol 1986;54(2):196-202.

Simon GE, Ludman EJ, Tutty S, et al. Telephone psychotherapy and telephone care management for primary care patients starting antidepressant treatment: a randomized controlled trial. JAMA 2004;292(8):935-42.

Simon GE, Ludman EJ, Rutter CM. Incremental benefit and cost of telephone care management and telephone psychotherapy for depression in primary care. Arch Gen Psychiatry 2009;66(10):1081-9.

Wilson PH. Combined pharmacological and behavioural treatment of depression. Behav Res Ther 1982;20(2):173-84.

Wilson PH. Comparative efficacy of behavioral and cognitive therapies of depression. Cognit Ther Res 1983;7(2):111-124

APPENDIX C: REVIEWER COMMENTS AND RESPONSES

Reviewer	Comment	Response
Question 1: Are the objectives, scope, and methods for this review clearly described?		
1	No – I can't follow the literature review here or in the text. KQ 1 involves evaluation of "brief therapies" which seem to be defined as 8 or fewer sessions.	We have added further explanation to both the Methods and Results sections of our overall approach and more explanation of what constitutes a "complex systematic review." We have also clearly delineated that, for the purposes of this review, ≤ 8 sessions are defined as "brief," 12 to 20 sessions are described as "standard," and psychotherapies of other durations are specifically designated.
	In general, I just don't get the Results for KQ1. I wonder if organizing your results by type of therapy might be more helpful. For example, "We identified X articles evaluating CBT: X were from the primary literature review and X were identified from the systematic reviews.	We have further clarified our overall approach and portions of KQ 1 to make apparent our structure of discussing systematic review findings prior to primary literature findings.
	Results: I have read this 3 times and still cannot follow the flow of literature. This needs to be clarified. Figure 2 also could be clarified by adding 2 boxes below the one describing the 2 SR's which shows how many articles come from each of the SR's and then connecting it to the very bottom box.	We have altered the literature flow figure to better indicate how we used the primary literature and systematic reviews.
	Nice summary and discussion.	Thank you.
	I think the important point that most of these studies involve women deserves more than a line in the limitations section. This is a huge issue for the VA. Were you able to tease out any gender sub-analyses from the SR's or the original articles?	We agree and have added consideration of this point to the discussion section. While we agree that a subanalysis would be interesting, we have not conducted such an analysis because the data are not adequate or appropriate, and AHRQ guidelines recommend against such analyses.
2	Unsure – Overall, the objectives, scope, and methods are clearly described. However, it is recommended that additional specificity be provided in references to "brief" versus "longer duration" psychotherapies throughout the manuscript, including the executive summary (e.g., p. 1, lines 14-15: "First, brief psychotherapies compared to longer duration psychotherapies had similar effect sizes.") The reference "longer duration" is often used in the report to refer to psychotherapy lengths that are still quite brief (e.g., 7-8+ sessions). Because this term is typically associated with psychotherapies of longer lengths (e.g., 12-16+ sessions), it would likely be helpful to be specific in such references to avoid confusion. Furthermore, there was a finding of a larger effect for the somewhat longer duration EBPs, though overlapping confidence intervals led to the conclusion that the evidence was inadequate to make a definitive determination. Thus, it is somewhat unclear what led to the statement above of similar effect sizes for brief vs. "longer" duration psychotherapies.	We have now clearly delineated that, for the purposes of this review, ≤ 8 sessions are defined as "brief," 12 to 20 sessions are described as "standard," and psychotherapies of other durations are specifically designated. We have also clarified our interpretation of overlapping confidence intervals for "brief" versus "standard" length psychotherapy.
3	Yes – No comment.	Acknowledged
4	Yes – The rationale for focusing the review on brief (8 or fewer sessions) is clear. The methodology employed in the review is well described. It was somewhat surprising that there was not a key question included that focused on a comparison of brief versus slightly longer standard psychotherapy (e.g., 12 to 16 sessions) in primary care. The authors note on Page 1, line 10 that there are guidelines recommending 12 to 16 one-hour sessions. For this reviewer, this number of sessions is the usual "gold standard" for clinical treatment and for clinical research in this area. Thus it would have been helpful to have a sense whether there is evidence that briefer treatment (8 or fewer sessions) is as efficacious as longer treatment.	The review that we originally proposed to conduct would have made this comparison. However, a variety of reasons contributed to our VA stakeholders recommending against conducting this comparison. Fortunately, the Cuijpers' systematic review addresses this comparison and allows us to make some tentative conclusions about comparative efficacy.
5	Yes – The objectives and scope are very clearly described and this review adheres nicely to its objectives and scope. The description of the search strategy (page 14) was somewhat confusing, particularly with regards to the selection of the specific dates to include in the Jan 2009-Aug 2010 search of MEDLINE, PsycINFO, Embase. After reading it a few times, I think I understand why those dates were chosen, but am still not entirely confident.	We have reworked this section to provide clarification on our search strategy.

Reviewer	Comment	Response
Question 2: Is there any indication of bias in our synthesis of the evidence?		
1	Not answered but no comments.	Acknowledged
2	No – no comment.	Acknowledged
3	No – no comment.	Acknowledged
4	No – This appears to be an exhaustive search of the literature, and the synthesis of the available data is excellent.	Thank you.
5	No – no comment.	Acknowledged
Question 3: Are there any studies of interest to the VA that we have overlooked?		
1	Not answered but also not addressed	Acknowledged
2	No – no comment.	Acknowledged
3	No – no comment.	Acknowledged
4	No – None that this reviewer is aware of.	Acknowledged
5	No – no comment.	Acknowledged
Question 4: Please write additional suggestions or comments below. If applicable, please indicate the page and line numbers from the draft report.		
1	On page 5 lines 6 and 7. 15 articles are described.	We have clarified the number of articles being described.
	Next, on page 5 line 16 is a description of findings from the systematic reviews of 6-16 sessions but I thought the focus was on brief interventions?	The reference to 6-16 sessions has been deleted so that the focus of this section of the Executive Summary is exclusively on brief psychotherapies.
	Line 21 then talks about a meta-analysis of 6 trials. Where did 6 come from?	This sentence was reworded to indicate that the 6 trials were a subset of CBT trials that we examined.
	Line 8 page 6 – What about the other systematic review? Any data on number of sessions from it?	The other systematic review was limited exclusively to brief psychotherapies, so no comparison could be made between brief psychotherapies and standard-length psychotherapies.
	Page 8, lines 2 and 3 contain information that should be presented earlier in the Results section (perhaps page 5 first paragraph). This limitation should still be discussed in the conclusions.	This information is now also presented early in the Results section of the Executive Summary.
	Methods: Page 14 lines 9 on – This paragraph needs to be clearer and for clarity, each search strategy should probably have its own paragraph. I believe lines 11-14 belong in the Results section.	Separate paragraphs have been created to enhance clarity, and the referenced lines have been moved to appropriate places in the Results section.
	Methods: Data Synthesis – Clarify what you mean in line 20 page 17. Which findings are you summarizing – the unique studies or the reviews findings?	We have clarified that we summarize in narrative form the systematic review findings.
	On page 22 line 5 the 2 systematic reviews are described and the authors identify 7 articles that are relevant to the review. Next, on page 24 line 1, the authors describe a systematic review including 34 studies but imply, not clearly however, that 14 of them contribute to the KQ addressed in this review. How did you get from 34 articles to the 9 articles described on page 23 and in Figure 2? How many came from the Cape review? The entire paragraph describing the Cape review needs to be clarified.	The reason for this discrepancy is that the Cuijpers review was described on page 22, while the Cape review was described on page 24. We have made changes throughout the document to more fully describe the "complex systematic review" that we conducted, including why we report on reviews that cover some articles that did not meet our inclusion criteria for individual studies (i.e., a systematic review could meet our inclusion criteria for systematic reviews even if not every article covered in a review met our inclusion criteria for primary literature).
	Page 25. Lines 3-6 are already in Methods.	This section has been modified to parallel our description results for the systematic review search.
	Lines 9-12 on page 25 are helpful.	Acknowledged
	Page 29 line 1. It would be helpful to begin, "Of the 15 unique studies, six studies…" so that it is clear where you are going with this paragraph.	Change made as suggested.

Reviewer	Comment	Response
1 (cont.)	Page 29 line 11—I would begin a new paragraph with, "The intervention…"	Change made as suggested.
	Page 30 line 17—Why 15 RCT's? I though you only found 8? Help! Why are you reporting the findings from their review when it does not address KQ1 dealing with brief therapies? This is confusing!	Please see above response for how we clarified this apparent discrepancy.
	Page 31 line 7—34 studies? You just talked for a few pages about how you got to 15. Clarify.	Please see above response for how we clarified this apparent discrepancy.
	Page 32—lines 3-9 need to be clarified. Perhaps using subtitles such as CBT or MBCT would be helpful?	We have altered the position of CBT in the initial sentence to help clarify that this paragraph is exclusively about CBT.
	Page 36 line 20—? 9 sessions?	We have changed "fewer than 9" to "≤ 8."
	If you have data on medical therapy among the controls in the 15 studies this would be very helpful. Were most of the controls treated with medicine or just followed? Since this is the comparison most people are interested in, it seems to me that it deserves more discussion	For the purposes of this review, we intentionally excluded trials that used standardized medication protocols (i.e., what we considered a separate active treatment condition). Many of the control groups were "usual care," which could possibly entail patients receiving medication, but usual care was highly variable.
2	The conclusion that brief EBPs are efficacious is somewhat tenuous, given the limited state of the research in this area and the limitations of many of the studies (e.g., many low quality studies, high heterogeneity, limited definition of usual care comparison groups, small effect sizes), methodology required for the review (pooled comparisons), and significant differences between the samples included in the reviewed studies and the Veteran population. While the report notes many of these limitations, it is recommended that the conclusion in the Discussion (p. 40, lines 2-3; "We conclude that brief psychotherapy is an efficacious treatment option for patients with depression in VA primary care settings") be qualified somewhat. Further, in the Cuijpers review, the finding of a significant effect for brief EBPs was only seen for studies in which patients were referred by their GP for treatment but not for those recruited through systematic screening. Given the magnitude of the differential effect, it may be worth noting this more directly in response to Question 1 in the Discussion. Moreover, while it may very well be that brief EBP is an efficacious treatment option for VA primary care settings, the reviewed studies were conducted overwhelmingly on non-Veterans. Perhaps more significant, many of the studies had diagnoses commonly seen in Veteran primary care patients as exclusionary criteria (e.g., substance abuse, psychosis, suicidality). This is worth explicitly noting in the context of discussing and perhaps qualifying the conclusions somewhat. There is brief, one-sentence mention in the Limitations section that the studies in the review was composed primarily middle-aged, Caucasian females, which does not seem sufficient.	We concur with many of these points and have qualified the statement. We have now commented on the differential effect between GP referral and systematic screening in the Discussion of KQ 1. We have more overtly acknowledged the limitations for the Veteran population, including the low representation of Veterans in the studies we reviewed, lack of comorbidity, and overrepresentation by middle-aged Caucasian females.
	It seems difficult to make highly meaningful interpretations of the results of many of the treatment group comparisons (e.g., brief EBP vs. usual care), since usual care was poorly described and variable in the reviewed studies. Furthermore, it is safe to assume that care as usual in many of most of the reviewed studies did not consist of evidence-based "care management," as is now implemented in most VA primary care settings. It would likely be valuable to note this in the Discussion.	We have commented on the VA's commitment to evidence-based care management in the Discussion. To our knowledge, the data remain out on whether VA's investment in evidence-based care management has in practice resulted in significantly better usual care than was received in the studies we reviewed.
	Given the lack of research comparing brief EBPs with full course EBPs, it is important that the implementation of brief EBPs not come at the expense or replacement of full course EBPs (which could occur due to local leadership perception that brief EBPs are effective and a desire for efficiency). The report notes that a comparison of brief EBPs with full course EBPs was not directly tested in the studies included in the review and suggests this, appropriately so, as an area of future inquiry. While direct comparison of brief vs. full course EBPs was not tested in the studies included in the review, it might be valuable to note the effect sizes commonly found in reviews of full course CBT and PST, or to consider this separately.	We sympathize with these concerns. After careful consideration, we have decided not to cite effect sizes for evidence-based psychotherapies from other reviews, as these effect sizes could be misleading should the reader compare them to the effect sizes we report for brief psychotherapy. Fortunately, the Cuijpers review makes this comparison in a subset of carefully selected trials, and we have elaborated on the caution warranted in interpreting their comparison because it is indirect and large CIs are involved.

Reviewer	Comment	Response
2 (cont.)	P. 40, lines 11-12: There does not seem to be sufficient evidence to support the conclusion that "broad training in mental health may not be necessary to provide these therapies." It is noted in the manuscript that some of the studies included therapists who were "graduate students, nurses, general practitioners, and other allied health professionals." It is further suggested that "Within the VA, a range of providers could be considered, including nurses, nurse practitioners, primary care physicians, social workers, and chaplains" to deliver brief EBPs. However, the inclusion of some non-MH providers in some studies does not seem sufficient for determining that individuals without background in mental health could deliver these treatments effectively (or as effectively) as mental health professionals, and there is no data to indicate the extent to which mental health training had an impact on, or moderated, outcomes. In fact, because the results were pooled across different provider types, it is quite possible that effects would have been higher if the treatments were delivered by mental health providers. It is also possible that there was not a significant effect for CBT or PST when delivered by non-MH providers. Were results of the studies available by provider-type? In addition, GPs and others noted above were identified in some of the PST studies; were these provider-types also included for CBT? Furthermore, VA patients are typically more complex and often have comorbidities (substance abuse, suicidality, psychosis) that were excluded in many of the reviewed studies and would often require a higher level professional to monitor and sometimes adapt treatment for. In addition, several of provider-types noted above are not locally credentialed to deliver brief EBPs in VHA. It is also worth noting that graduate students and clinical social workers (as well as nurses with background in mental health) are considered mental health providers in VHA and often deliver EBPs, along with psychologists and psychiatrists.	We have tempered our statements regarding necessary training and emphasized the need for more research on the use of "non–mental health professionals" to provide brief EBPs.
	EBPs have often been shown to more efficacious in treating major depression than dysthymia. It may be useful to break out results for different types of depression to the extent that this is possible (i.e., if there are sufficient number of studies/participants without mixed diagnostic groups).	We have now included in our KQ 1 Results information from the Cuijpers review on MDD versus "other" diagnoses.
	The finding of Cape of a large effect size for treatment of anxiety is interesting and significantly higher than the effect-sizes for mixed anxiety and depression and depression only. Although anxiety is beyond the scope of the current review, it would be interesting to know what type of anxiety this included (e.g., generalized anxiety or other specific forms of anxiety?). Might this finding be an artifact of the research (e.g., smaller sample size), rather than the being a true differential effect for this condition?	We now note that "anxiety" refers predominantly to diagnoses of panic and generalized anxiety disorder. Although we do not expound on this finding because it is beyond the scope of this review, we would caution interpretation of the difference due to the indirect comparison methodology, but we would also suggest that the finding may represent a true difference and is of value as a hypothesis generating finding.
3	This is a well done review. Methods used to identify studies were appropriate. Decision to review previously published reviews and add additional studies not included in those reviews seems a good one.	Thank you.
	Tables 3 and 4 do a nice job of summarizing the included studies – they are well organized and easy to understand.	
	The moderate effect size in relation to usual care was noted. I wonder if an analysis could be done to see if there is an association between depression severity and effect size. I would hypothesize that psychotherapy would be most effective for those with moderate symptoms, less effective for those with mild symptoms, and least effective (at least as monotherapy) for those with severe symptoms. It would be useful to know if the literature supports targeting any subgroups of patients as the best candidates for brief psychotherapy.	Such an analysis was not possible with the data obtained from the primary literature. However, we have added as a limitation our inability to answer this question.
4	Given the large numbers of older veterans receiving care in the VA system, some mention of acceptability and efficacy of brief psychotherapies in older adults would help the discussion. Several of their cited studies include or are entirely focused on older adults, so some specific comment on this population would help. This is particularly relevant since older white males have among the highest rates of completed suicide, and studies have shown that a large proportion of completed suicide victims in this age group have recently seen a primary care physician. In sum, the inclusion of a discussion of the relevance of depression in older veterans would add much to the report.	The 2 out of 15 studies that contained elderly participant samples are now separately examined in the Results. Also, additional mention on lack of data in Veteran samples (or male/elderly samples) is now made in the Discussion.

Reviewer	Comment	Response
5	This is a very clearly written report that does a nice job utilizing the available research literature to address the key questions it sets out to answer. The ability of this review to identify and outline some shortcomings in our current knowledge base will provide an important foundation for future research on brief psychotherapies for depression and the use of psychotherapy in primary care settings. A study characteristic that is not addressed in this review, but may be useful to consider, or at least mention, is treatment dropout rate.	Thank you. We have revised a column heading in Table 4 to "Therapy completed" to indicate the number patients retained in the treatment condition (i.e., those that did not dropout).
	The remainder of my comments consist of minor wording suggestions or clarifications:	
	Throughout the document, the word "Veteran" should be consistently capitalized. I would also suggest consistency in whether quality of life has hyphens between the words (i.e. quality-of-life) or not (i.e. quality of life).	"Veteran" and "Veterans" have been capitalized throughout.

The phrase "quality of life" appears with hyphens when used as a unit modifier, as in "quality-of-life measures." Most instances in the report are not this usage, so we have left those without hyphens. |
	P 7, line 17 and p 40, line 11: the suggestion that "broad" training in mental health may not be necessary. I would guess that all of the other non-mental health specialists being discussed here probably do in fact have "broad" training in mental health, but may not have "extensive" or "specialized" training in mental health, so there may be a more accurate way to capture what you are trying to say here.	We have tempered our statements to more strictly state what we found in the review and to emphasize the need for more research on the use of "non-mental health professionals" to provide brief EBPs.
	Page 11, line 7 – suggest using "intensive" rather than "demanding"	Changed as suggested.
	Page 11, lines 14-17 – the wording of this sentence is awkward and therefore does not convey the importance of this review as clearly and strongly as possible.	The sentence has been split into two sentences and reworded.
	Page 21 and 22 – in the description of the Cuijpers review, p21, line 17 refers to 15 studies, but p 22, line 5 says, "Of the 16 trials…"	16 was a mistake; we have changed to 15.
	Page 24, lines 13-14 – the sentence about what countries the studies were conducted in is confusing. Throughout most of this paragraph the authors are talking about the "14 depression studies" but then say that only one in seven were conducted in the US. Does this mean 2 of the 14 were conducted in the US?	Yes, that is what was meant. We have reworded the sentence to enhance clarity.
	Table 3: Does "most distal follow up" time period refer to the length of time between baseline and most distal follow up or between the end of treatment and the most distal follow up? It would be helpful to clarify this in the table (even if it is described in the text).	A footnote has been added to the table for clarification.
	Table 4: I would suggest moving the sample size to Table 3, since it seems more like a characteristic of the study than of the intervention. I would also suggest using "intervention n" or "treatment n" (and then define what this means) for that column rather than "completed n" and "control n". It would make a sense to keep the completion rates for the intervention arm as a column in Table 4. The therapy intensity column of Table 4 is a little difficult to digest. Perhaps having separate columns for session length and frequency of sessions would make it easier to understand?	We have split the therapy intensity column into two columns as suggested and have changed the column heading for "completed n." We concur with the reviewer's sentiment that sample size is more a characteristic of the study than the intervention, but we decided not to move this information in order to consolidate information in Table 4 and to cut down on clutter in Table 3.
	Page 29, lines 17-18 – I would suggest re-wording this sentence to something like, "Follow-up duration was less than 6 months for 7 studies 6 months or greater for 8 studies."	Sentence has been reworded as suggested.
	Page 29, line 21 refers to the fact that only 2 study samples included any Veteran representation. It might be helpful to add a little more detail about what proportion of the samples were Veterans in those 2 studies, or if they were studies specifically of Veterans, etc.	Additional detail has been added here and throughout the report.
	In the Cuijpers review, was the ES for ≤ 6 sessions smaller than it was for interventions that included more than 6 sessions? Page 31, line 3, reports that brief psychotherapies had a small but significant positive effect for treatment of depression in primary care – did Cuijpers examine whether this ES of -0.25 was statistically smaller than that for the full range of studies they looked at (ES -0.31 reported on page 30, line 19)?	The Cuijpers review does make a comparison between ≤ 6 sessions and > 6 sessions, and they did not find a statistically significant difference. We report these findings in KQ 2 because the comparison between brief and standard-duration psychotherapies is the focus of KQ 2.
	In the Cape meta analysis, is the ES of -0.21 reported on page 31, line 11 referring to the combined ES for depression AND mixed anxiety and depression?	Yes. We have clarified by identifying the different diagnostic categories from the outset of this paragraph and by pointing out that the authors combined diagnostic categories for some of their analyses.

Reviewer	Comment	Response
5 (cont.)	Page 31, lines 16-18 – The sentences describing the ES for brief psychotherapies specifically for depression is somewhat contradictory. On the one hand, the authors report a "slightly smaller" effect for PST over usual GP care (as compared to the effect for CBT over usual GP care), but then report "no significant differences in efficacy between CBT and PST. This could possibly be re-worded to say that the ES was slightly smaller, but not significantly different, for PST, but even this is still somewhat contradictory. (i.e. if it's not statistically significantly smaller, can it be called smaller?)	The issue here is that at the p = 0.05 level, CBT demonstrated statistical significance and PST did not. Because there was no statistically significant difference between CBT and PST, because CBT narrowly demonstrated statistical significance at the p = 0.05 level, and because PST would demonstrate statistical significance at a slightly more lenient p level (e.g., p = 0.06 or 0.07), we feel that it would be misleading to draw too much attention to the fact that CBT achieved significance (narrowly) at the arbitrary 0.05 mark and PST did not (narrowly). We have reworded this sentence to remove the contradiction.
	Page 32, line 11: I would suggest replacing "judged to" with "rated as"	Changed as suggested.
	Page 32, line 14: Do you want to add (n=1) after the word antidepressant?	Yes, changed as suggested.
	Page 33, line 9: I am unsure of exactly what the term "irregular comparator condition" means.	We have clarified this sentence by replacing the term "irregular comparator" with a more accurate description of the control condition.
	Figure 3: In the labels under the Sd diff in means and 95% CI, do the authors intentionally use "Favours" in stead of "Favors"?	The British spelling has been changed to "Favors."
	Page 35, lines 12-14: Stating that "These results are consistent with both Cape's and Cuijpers' conclusion that PST is an efficacious option for the treatment of depression." may be slightly overstating it, since one of the 2 studies did find a difference and the other did not, especially since the better quality trial did not find that PST improved outcomes.	We have altered a sentence to clarify that although the Mynors-Wallis study found PST+Med no better than Med alone, they also found that PST alone was equally as effective as Med alone. On this basis, we still conclude that the results are consistent with the conclusion that PST is an efficacious treatment option.
	Page 37, lines 10-13: The authors could put the number of studies with each type of provider in parentheses (e.g. n=3), as they did on page 32 (lines 11-14)	We retained the sentence structure to avoid ambiguity (e.g., n = 3 could be interpreted as 3 studies or as 3 psychologists).
	On page 38, I would suggest adding a sentence after line 3 noting that the numbers of studies in each sub-group were too small to conduct quantitative analyses of provider type, individual vs. group, telephone vs. in person or treatment intensity. Though this is fairly obvious, it would make it explicit and also make it consistent with other sections of the review in which similar decisions were made.	Changed as suggested.
	On page 40, line 1-2, I would suggest saying more about the statement, "However, usual care may represent a more potent control condition than placebo controls used in antidepressant trials." What do the authors mean? What makes them think this could be the case?	We have expounded on this statement to describe that it may be the case that usual care is more effective than placebo control because patients treated with usual care are receiving what is intended to be an active treatment and could even be a "best practice" treatment.
	Page 40, line 14 – I would suggest changing the phrase "appropriate training and supervision" to something like "training and supervision specific to the intervention being conducted". Since many studies do not give much detail about the training provided, and since we really don't have data that tells us how much or what kind of training is needed to implement these interventions, I'm not sure it can be deemed "appropriate" (or inappropriate) based on the information provided in each study.	Changed as suggested. We have also tempered our statements to more strictly state what we found in the review and to emphasize the need for more research on the use of "non–mental health professionals" to provide brief EBPs.
	Page 41, line 16 – suggest using the term "screened" rather than "selected" in reference to identifying patients who would be appropriate for brief psychotherapy	Changed as suggested.
	Page 42, line 11 – I would suggest replacing "appropriate" (in reference to the quantitative synthesis methods) with something like "rigorous" or "robust" to convey that you not only chose analyses that were appropriate, but that you chose the best available methods. This is indeed a strength of this review and even that slight wording change conveys that in a stronger manner.	Changed as suggested.

APPENDIX D: EXCLUDED STUDIES

All studies listed below were reviewed in their full-text version and excluded for the reason indicated. An alphabetical reference list follows the table.

Reference	Population not appropriate	Intervention not of interest	Comparator not appropriate	Not SR or RCT	> 8 therapy sessions planned	Main outcome not of interest
Abbass-Allen, 2006 (535)	X					
Abraham, 1992 (656)					X	
Alexopoulis, 2003 (657)					X	
Anonymous, 2010 (733)				X		
Arean, 1993 (658)					X	
Barrera, 1979 (685)			X			
Bedi, 2000 (686)			X			
Bee, 2010 (708)	X					
Bell, 2009 (458)	X					
Beutler, 1987 (659)	X				X	
Boer, 2005 (575)	X					
Bortolotti, 2008 (71)		X				
Campbell, 1992 (660)						X
Catalan, 1991 (661)	X					
Ciechanowski, 2004 (662)			X			
Coelho, 2007 (447)	X					
Cole, 2008 (74)	X					
Comas-Diaz (702)			X			
Cuijpers, 2008 (469)	X					
Cuijpers, 2010 (31)		X				
Cuijpers, 2010 (467)		X				
Cuijpers, 2007 (137)	X					
Cuijpers, 2008 (76)				X		
Cuijpers, 2007 (462)	X					
de Mello, 2005 (355)					X	
Dhooper, 1993 (736)		X				
Doorenbos, 2005 (663)	X					
Dozios, 2009 (709)					X	
Driessen, 2010 (510)	X					
Ekers, 2008 (345)	X					
Fleming, 1980 (687)			X			
Floyd, 2004 (665)					X	
Fry, 1984 (737)					X	

Reference	Population not appropriate	Intervention not of interest	Comparator not appropriate	Not SR or RCT	> 8 therapy sessions planned	Main outcome not of interest
Fuchs, 1997 (688)		X				
Gardner, 1981 (689)			X			
Godbole, 1973 (667)	X					
Hamdan-Mansauer, 2009 (711)					X	
Haringsma, 2006 (668)					X	
Hegerl, 2010 (713)					X	
Hogg, 1988 (744)			X			
Holland, 2009 (714)	X	X				
Hsu, 2009 (715)						X
Huffziger, 2009 (716)	X					
Hynninen, 2010 (718)	X					
Jarvik, 1982 (669)			X			
Kanter, 2010 (719)	X				X	
Katon, 2004 (672)	X					
Konnert, 2009 (720)	X					
Kotova, 2005 (342)	X				X	
LaPointe, 1980 (748)	X	X				
Latour, 1994 (738)	X	X				
Lichtenberg, 1996 (739)	X					
Lynch, 2010 (33)	X	X				
Mackin, 2005 (177)		X				
Mazzuchelli, 2009 (368)			X			
McCurren, 1999 (673)		X				
McKnight, 1992 (740)		X				
McNaughton, 2009 (21)		X				
Miranda, 2003 (691)			X			
Mohr, 2008 (498)		X				
Montgomery, 2010 (372)	X					
Mynor-Wallis, 1997 (674)	X					
Nezu, 1989 (678)	X				X	
Nezu, 2003 (677)	X					
Oranta, 2010 (722)	X					
Pace, 1993 (704)	X					
Parker, 2007 (517)				X		
Pecheur, 1984 (706)	X		X			
Peden, 2000 (697)	X					
Peng, 2009 (19)					X	

Reference	Population not appropriate	Intervention not of interest	Comparator not appropriate	Not SR or RCT	> 8 therapy sessions planned	Main outcome not of interest
Petersen, 2010 (734)	X					
Pigeon, 2009 (723)	X					
Powers, 2009 (358)	X					
Reynolds, 1999 (680)	X					
Sallis, 1983 (741)					X	
Serfaty, 2009 (724)					X	
Shaw, 1977 (698)		X				
Sirey, 2005 (692)		X				
Stulz, 2010 (728)				X		
Taylor, 1977 (707)			X			
Thompson, 1984 (742)				X		
Thompson, 1987 (743)					X	
Tsang, 2008 (93)		X				
Uebelacker, 2009 (729)				X		
Unutzer, 2002 (681)			X			
Van Calker, 2009 (730)	X					
Watkins, 2009 (693)		X				
Watkins, 2009 (732)		X				
Warmerdam, 2010 (731)		X				
Wierzbicki, 1987 (746)			X			
Wood, 1997 (682)	X					
Yang, 2009 (696)	X					
Zerhusen, 1991 (683)					X	

LIST OF EXCLUDED STUDIES

Abbass Allan A, Hancock Jeffrey T, Henderson J, et al. Short-term psychodynamic psychotherapies for common mental disorders. Cochrane Database of Systematic Reviews 2006(4).

Abraham IL, Neundorfer MM, Currie LJ. Effects of group interventions on cognition and depression in nursing home residents. Nurs Res 1992;41(4):196-202.

Alexopoulos GS, Raue P, Arean P. Problem-solving therapy versus supportive therapy in geriatric major depression with executive dysfunction. Am J Geriatr Psychiatry 2003;11(1):46-52.

Anonymous. Cognitive Behavioral Therapy Effective for Depressed Elderly. J Natl Med Assoc 2010;102(4):358.

Arean PA, Perri MG, Nezu AM, et al. Comparative effectiveness of social problem-solving therapy and reminiscence therapy as treatments for depression in older adults. J Consult Clin Psychol 1993;61(6):1003-10.

Barrera M, Jr. An evaluation of a brief group therapy for depression. J Consult Clin Psychol 1979;47(2):413-5.

Bedi N, Chilvers C, Churchill R, et al. Assessing effectiveness of treatment of depression in primary care. Partially randomised preference trial. Br J Psychiatry 2000;177:312-8.

Bee PE, Bower P, Gilbody S, et al. Improving health and productivity of depressed workers: a pilot randomized controlled trial of telephone cognitive behavioral therapy delivery in workplace settings. Gen Hosp Psychiatry 2010;32(3):337-40.

Bell AC, D'Zurilla TJ. Problem-solving therapy for depression: A meta-analysis. Clin Psychol Rev 2009;29(4):348-353.

Beutler LE, Scogin F, Kirkish P, et al. Group cognitive therapy and alprazolam in the treatment of depression in older adults. J Consult Clin Psychol 1987;55(4):550-6.

Boer Peter CAM, Wiersma D, Russo S, et al. Paraprofessionals for anxiety and depressive disorders. Cochrane Database of Systematic Reviews 2005(2).

Bortolotti B, Menchetti M, Bellini F, et al. Psychological interventions for major depression in primary care: a meta-analytic review of randomized controlled trials. Gen Hosp Psychiatry 2008;30(4):293-302.

Campbell JM. Treating depression in well older adults: use of diaries in cognitive therapy. Issues Ment Health Nurs 1992;13(1):19-29.

Catalan J, Gath DH, Anastasiades P, et al. Evaluation of a brief psychological treatment for emotional disorders in primary care. Psychol Med 1991;21(4):1013-8.

Ciechanowski P, Wagner E, Schmaling K, et al. Community-integrated home-based depression treatment in older adults: a randomized controlled trial. JAMA 2004;291(13):1569-77.

Coelho HF, Canter PH, Ernst E. Mindfulness-based cognitive therapy: Evaluating current evidence and informing future research. J Consult Clin Psychol 2007;75(6):1000-1005.

Cole MG. Brief interventions to prevent depression in older subjects: a systematic review of feasibility and effectiveness. Am J Geriatr Psychiatry 2008;16(6):435-43.

Comas-Diaz L. Effects of cognitive and behavioral group treatment on the depressive symptomatology of Puerto Rican women. J Consult Clin Psychol 1981;49(5):627-32.

Cuijpers P, van Straten A, Andersson G, et al. Psychotherapy for depression in adults: A meta-analysis of comparative outcome studies. J Consult Clin Psychol 2008;76(6):909-922.

Cuijpers P, van Straten A, Bohlmeijer E, et al. The effects of psychotherapy for adult depression are overestimated: a meta-analysis of study quality and effect size. Psychol Med 2010;40(2):211-23.

Cuijpers P, van Straten A, Schuurmans J, et al. Psychotherapy for chronic major depression and dysthymia: A meta-analysis. Clin Psychol Rev 2010;30(1):51-62.

Cuijpers P, van Straten A, Warmerdam L. Problem solving therapies for depression: a meta-analysis. Eur Psychiatry 2007;22(1):9-15.

Cuijpers P, van Straten A, Warmerdam L, et al. Psychological treatment of depression: a meta-analytic database of randomized studies. BMC Psychiatry 2008;8:36. Available at: (http://www.psychotherapy-rcts.org/index.php?id=3). Accessed November 10, 2010.

Cuijpers P, van Straten FSA. Psychological treatments of subthreshold depression: A meta-analytic review. Acta Psychiatr Scand 2007;115(6):434-441.

de Mello MF, de Jesus Mari J, Bacaltchuk J, et al. A systematic review of research findings on the efficacy of interpersonal therapy for depressive disorders. Eur Arch Psychiatry Clin Neurosci 2005;255(2):75-82.

Dhooper S, Green S, Huff M, et al. Efficacy of a group approach to reducing depression in nursing home elderly residents. Journal of Gerontological Social Work 1993;20(3/4):87-100.

Doorenbos A, Given B, Given C, et al. Reducing symptom limitations: a cognitive behavioral intervention randomized trial. Psychooncology 2005 ;14(7) :574-84.

Dozois DJ, Bieling PJ, Patelis-Siotis I, et al. Changes in self-schema structure in cognitive therapy for major depressive disorder: a randomized clinical trial. J Consult Clin Psychol 2009 ;77(6) :1078-88.

Driessen E, Cuijpers P, de Maat SCM, et al. The efficacy of short-term psychodynamic psychotherapy for depression: A meta-analysis. Clin Psychol Rev 2010;30(1):25-36.

Ekers D, Richards D, Gilbody S. A meta-analysis of randomized trials of behavioural treatment of depression. Psychological Medicine: A Journal of Research in Psychiatry and the Allied Sciences 2008;38(5):611-623.

Fleming BM, Thornton DW. Coping skills training as a component in the short-term treatment of depression. J Consult Clin Psychol 1980;48(5):652-4.

Floyd M, Scogin F, McKendree-Smith NL, et al. Cognitive therapy for depression: a comparison of individual psychotherapy and bibliotherapy for depressed older adults. Behav Modif 2004;28(2):297-318.

Fry P. Cognitive Training and Cognitive-Behavioral Variables in the Treatment of Depression in the Elderly. Clin Gerontol 1984;3(1):25-44.

Fuchs CZ, Rehm LP. A self-control behavior therapy program for depression. J Consult Clin Psychol 1977;45(2):206-15.

Gardner P, Oei TP. Depression and self-esteem: an investigation that used behavioral and cognitive approaches to the treatment of clinically depressed clients. J Clin Psychol 1981;37(1):128-35.

Godbole A, Verinis JS. Brief psychotherapy in the treatment of emotional disorders in physically ill geriatric patients. Gerontologist 1974;14(2):143-8.

Hamdan-Mansour AM, Puskar K, Bandak AG. Effectiveness of cognitive-behavioral therapy on depressive symptomatology, stress and coping strategies among Jordanian university students. Issues Ment Health Nurs 2009;30(3):188-96.

Haringsma R, Engels GI, Cuijpers P, et al. Effectiveness of the Coping With Depression (CWD) course for older adults provided by the community-based mental health care system in the Netherlands: a randomized controlled field trial. Int Psychogeriatr 2006;18(2):307-25.

Hegerl U, Hautzinger M, Mergl R, et al. Effects of pharmacotherapy and psychotherapy in depressed primary-care patients: a randomized, controlled trial including a patients' choice arm. Int J Neuropsychopharmacol 2010;13(1):31-44.

Hogg J, Deffenbacher J. A comparison of cognitive and interpersonal-process group therapies in the treatment of depression among college students. Journal of Counseling Psychology 1988;35(3):304-310.

Holland JM, Currier JM, Gallagher-Thompson D. Outcomes from the Resources for Enhancing Alzheimer's Caregiver Health (REACH) program for bereaved caregivers. Psychol Aging 2009;24(1):190-202.

Hsu YC, Wang JJ. Physical, affective, and behavioral effects of group reminiscence on depressed institutionalized elders in Taiwan. Nurs Res 2009;58(4):294-9.

Huffziger S, Kuehner C. Rumination, distraction, and mindful self-focus in depressed patients. Behav Res Ther 2009;47(3):224-30.

Hynninen MJ, Bjerke N, Pallesen S, et al. A randomized controlled trial of cognitive behavioral therapy for anxiety and depression in COPD. Respir Med 2010;104(7):986-94.

Jarvik LF, Mintz J, Steuer J, et al. Treating geriatric depression: a 26-week interim analysis. J Am Geriatr Soc 1982;30(11):713-7.

Kanter JW, Santiago-Rivera AL, Rusch LC, et al. Initial outcomes of a culturally adapted behavioral activation for Latinas diagnosed with depression at a community clinic. Behav Modif 2010;34(2):120-44.

Katon WJ, Von Korff M, Lin EH, et al. The Pathways Study: a randomized trial of collaborative care in patients with diabetes and depression. Arch Gen Psychiatry 2004;61(10):1042-9.

Konnert C, Dobson K, Stelmach L. The prevention of depression in nursing home residents: a randomized clinical trial of cognitive-behavioral therapy. Aging Ment Health 2009;13(2):288-99.

Kotova E. A meta-analysis of Interpersonal Psychotherapy. ProQuest Information & Learning; 2005.

LaPointe K, Rimm D. Cognitive, assertive, and insight-oriented group therapies in the treatment of reactive depression in women. Psychotherapy: Theory, Research and Practice 1980;17:312-321.

Latour D, Cappeliez P. Pretherapy training for group cognitive therapy with depressed older adults. Canadian Journal on Aging 1994;13(2):221-235.

Lichtenberg P. Behavioral Treatment of Depression in Predominantly African-American Medical Patients. Clin Gerontol 1996;17(2):15-33.

Lynch D, Laws KR, McKenna PJ. Cognitive behavioural therapy for major psychiatric disorder: does it really work? A meta-analytical review of well-controlled trials. Psychol Med 2010;40(1):9-24.

Mackin RS, Arean PA. Evidence-based psychotherapeutic interventions for geriatric depression. Psychiatr Clin North Am 2005;28(4):805-20, vii-viii.

Mazzucchelli T, Kane R, Rees C. Behavioral activation treatments for depression in adults: A meta-analysis and review. Clinical Psychology: Science and Practice 2009;16(4):383-411.

McCurren C, Dowe D, Rattle D, et al. Depression among nursing home elders: testing an intervention strategy. Appl Nurs Res 1999;12(4):185-95.

McKnight D, Nelson-Gray R, Barnhill J. Dexametnasone test and response to cognitive therapy and antidepressant medication. Behavior Therapy 1992;23(1):99-111.

McNaughton JL. Brief interventions for depression in primary care: a systematic review. Can Fam Physician 2009;55(8):789-96.

Miranda J, Chung JY, Green BL, et al. Treating depression in predominantly low-income young minority women: a randomized controlled trial. JAMA 2003;290(1):57-65.

Mohr DC, Vella L, Hart S, et al. The effect of telephone-administered psychotherapy on symptoms of depression and attrition: A meta-analysis. Clinical Psychology: Science and Practice 2008;15(3):243-253.

Montgomery EC, Kunik ME, Wilson N, et al. Can paraprofessionals deliver cognitive-behavioral therapy to treat anxiety and depressive symptoms? Bull Menninger Clin 2010;74(1):45-62.

Mynors-Wallis L, Davies I, Gray A, et al. A randomised controlled trial and cost analysis of problem-solving treatment for emotional disorders given by community nurses in primary care. Br J Psychiatry 1997;170:113-9.

Nezu AM, Nezu CM, Felgoise SH, et al. Project Genesis: assessing the efficacy of problem-solving therapy for distressed adult cancer patients. J Consult Clin Psychol 2003;71(6):1036-48.

Nezu AM, Perri MG. Social problem-solving therapy for unipolar depression: an initial dismantling investigation. J Consult Clin Psychol 1989;57(3):408-13.

Oranta O, Luutonen S, Salokangas RK, et al. The outcomes of interpersonal hristian on depressive symptoms and distress after myocardial infarction. Nord J Psychiatry 2010;64(2):78-86.

Pace T, Dixon D. Changes in depressive self-schemata and depressive symptoms following cognitive therapy. Journal of Counseling Psychology 1993;40(3):288-294.

Parker G, Fletcher K. Treating depression with the evidence-based psychotherapies: A critique of the evidence. Acta Psychiatr Scand 2007;115(5):352-359.

Pecheur D, Edwards K. A comparison of secular and religious versions of cognitive therapy with depressed hristian college students. Journal of Psychology and Theology 1984;12(1):45-54.

Peden AR, Hall LA, Rayens MK, et al. Reducing negative thinking and depressive symptoms in college women. J Nurs Scholarsh 2000;32(2):145-51.

Peng XD, Huang CQ, Chen LJ, et al. Cognitive behavioural therapy and reminiscence techniques for the treatment of depression in the elderly: a systematic review. J Int Med Res 2009;37(4):975-82.

Petersen T, Pava J, Burchin J, et al. The role of cognitive-behavioral therapy and fluoxetine in prevention of recurrence of major depressive disorder. Cognit Ther Res 2010;34:13-23.

Pigeon WR, May PE, Perlis ML, et al. The effect of interpersonal psychotherapy for depression on insomnia symptoms in a cohort of women with sexual abuse histories. J Trauma Stress 2009;22(6):634-8.

Powers MB, Zum Vörde Sive Vörding MB, Emmelkamp PMG. Acceptance and commitment therapy: A meta-analytic review. Psychother Psychosom 2009;78(2):73-80.

Reynolds CF, 3rd, Miller MD, Pasternak RE, et al. Treatment of bereavement-related major depressive episodes in later life: a controlled study of acute and continuation treatment with nortriptyline and interpersonal psychotherapy. Am J Psychiatry 1999;156(2):202-8.

Sallis J, Lichstein K, Clarkson A, et al. Anxiety and depression management for the elderly. Stalgeitis, Sinternational Journal of Behavioral Geriatrics 1983;1(4):3-12.

Serfaty MA, Haworth D, Blanchard M, et al. Clinical effectiveness of individual cognitive behavioral therapy for depressed older people in primary care: a randomized controlled trial. Arch Gen Psychiatry 2009;66(12):1332-40.

Shaw BF. Comparison of cognitive therapy and behavior therapy in the treatment of depression. J Consult Clin Psychol 1977 ;45(4) :543-51.

Sirey JA, Bruce ML, Alexopoulos GS. The Treatment Initiation Program: an intervention to improve depression outcomes in older adults. Am J Psychiatry 2005;162(1):184-6.

Stulz N, Thase ME, Klein DN, et al. Differential effects of treatments for chronic depression: a latent growth model reanalysis. J Consult Clin Psychol 2010;78(3):409-19.

Taylor F, Marshall W. Experimental analysis of a cognitive-behavioral therapy for depression Cognit Ther Res 1977;1(1):59-72.

Thompson L. Efficacy of psychotherapy in the treatment of Advances in behavior research and therapy 1984;6(2):127-139.

Thompson L, Gallagher D, Breckenridge J. Comparative effectiveness of psychotherapy for depressed elders. Journal of Consulting and Clinical Pyshcology 1987;55(3):385-390.

Tsang HW, Chan EP, Cheung WM. Effects of mindful and non-mindful exercises on people with depression: a systematic review. Br J Clin Psychol 2008;47(Pt 3):303-22.

Uebelacker LA, Weisberg RB, Haggarty R, et al. Adapted behavior therapy for persistently depressed primary care patients: an open trial. Behav Modif 2009;33(3):374-95.

Unutzer J, Katon W, Callahan CM, et al. Collaborative care management of late-life depression in the primary care setting: a randomized controlled trial. JAMA 2002;288(22):2836-45.

van Calker D, Zobel I, Dykierek P, et al. Time course of response to antidepressants: predictive value of early improvement and effect of additional psychotherapy. J Affect Disord 2009;114(1-3):243-53.

Warmerdam L, van Straten A, Jongsma J, et al. Online cognitive behavioral therapy and problem-solving therapy for depressive symptoms: Exploring mechanisms of change. J Behav Ther Exp Psychiatry 2010;41(1):64-70.

Watkins ER, Baeyens CB, Read R. Concreteness training reduces dysphoria: proof-of-principle for repeated cognitive bias modification in depression. J Abnorm Psychol 2009;118(1):55-64.

Watkins ER, Moberly NJ. Concreteness training reduces dysphoria: a pilot proof-of-principle study. Behav Res Ther 2009;47(1):48-53.

Wierzbicki M, Bartlett T. The efficacy of group and individual cognitive therapy for mild depression. Cognit Ther Res 1987;11(3):337-342.

Wood BC, Mynors-Wallis LM. Problem-solving therapy in palliative care. Palliat Med 1997;11(1):49-54.

Yang TT, Hsiao FH, Wang KC, et al. The effect of psychotherapy added to pharmacotherapy on cortisol responses in outpatients with major depressive disorder. J Nerv Ment Dis 2009;197(6):401-6.

Zerhusen JD, Boyle K, Wilson W. Out of the darkness: group cognitive therapy for depressed elderly. J Psychosoc Nurs Ment Health Serv 1991;29(9):16-21.

APPENDIX E: ACRONYMS AND ABBREVIATIONS

ACT	acceptance and commitment therapy
AE	adverse effects
BDI-II	Beck Depression Inventory-II
CBASP	cognitive behavioral analysis system of psychotherapy
CBT	cognitive behavioral therapy
CES-D	Center for Epidemiologic Studies-Depression
CI	confidence interval
CM	care management
DBT	dialectical behavioral therapy
DHP	Diabetes Health Profile
DIS	Diagnostic Interview Schedule
DSM-IV	Diagnostic and Statistical Manual of Mental Disorders
FAP	functional analytic psychotherapy
GP	general practitioner
HAM-D	Hamilton Depression Scale
HRSD	Hamilton Rating Scale for Depression
HSLC-D	Headache Specific Locus of Control-Depression
IPT	interpersonal therapy
LOCF	last observation carried forward
MBCT	mindfulness-based cognitive therapy
MDD	major depressive disorder
MDE	major depressive episode
MH	mental health
MMPI-D	Minnesota Multiphasic Personality Inventory-Depression
MMSE	Mini Mental State Examination
MOS-D	Medical Outcomes Study-Depression

N or n	number
NA	not applicable
NNT	number needed to treat
NR	not reported
NS or ns	not significant
OR	odds ratio
p	probability
PC	primary care
PFT	problem-focused therapy
PHQ	Patient Health Questionnaire
PRIME-MD	Primary Care Evaluation of Mental Disorders
PST	problem-solving treatment
PTSD	posttraumatic stress disorder
RCT	randomized controlled trial
RDC	Research Diagnostic Criteria
Rx	medicine prescription
SADS-L	Schedule for Affective Disorders and Schizophrenia-Lifetime Version
SCAN	Schedules for Clinical Assessment in Neuropsychiatry
SCL	Symptom Checklist
SD	standard deviation
SE	standard error
ST	standard treatment
TAU	treatment as usual
vs	versus
WHOQOL	World Health Organization Quality of Life
wk	week or weeks
WLC	waitlist control
yr	year or years

www.ingramcontent.com/pod-product-compliance
Lightning Source LLC
Chambersburg PA
CBHW081605170526
45166CB00009B/2836